I'm Too Young To Have a Heart Attack

How to Order:

Quantity discounts are available from the publisher, Prima Publishing, P.O. Box 1260CAS, Rocklin, CA 95677; telephone (916) 624-5718. On your letterhead include information concerning the intended use of the books and the number of books you wish to purchase.

U.S. Bookstores and Libraries: Please submit all orders to St. Martin's Press, 175 Fifth Avenue, New York, NY 10010; telephone (212) 674-5151.

I'M TOO YOUNG TO HAVE A HEART ATTACK

Jim Castelli

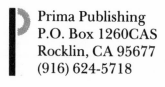 Prima Publishing
P.O. Box 1260CAS
Rocklin, CA 95677
(916) 624-5718

Copy Editing by Emily Hutchinson
Production by Rosaleen Bertolino, Bookman Productions
Typography by Janet Hansen, Alphatype
Interior design by Judith Levinson
Jacket design by The Dunlavey Studio
Author photo by Jayne Castelli

Prima Publishing
Rocklin, CA

Library of Congress Cataloging-in-Publication Data

Castelli, Jim.
  I'm too young to have a heart attack / Jim Castelli.
    p. cm.
  Includes bibliographical references.
  ISBN 1-55958-026-7
    1. Castelli, Jim—Health. 2. Heart—Infarction—
Patients—United States—Biography. 3. Journalists—
United States—Biography.
  I. Title.
RC685.I6C373   1990
362.1'96123'0092—dc20
[B]   90-36216
                                  CIP

90 91 92 93 RRD 10 9 8 7 6 5 4 3 2 1

Printed in the United States of America

For Jayne, Matt, and Dan

ACKNOWLEDGMENTS

I'd like to thank my agent, Jeff Herman, and his assistant, Deborah Adams, for helping me put more of myself into this book, and Jim Metcalf for his foreword and encouragement. I'd also like to thank the dozens of people—hospital staff, friends and neighbors, and fellow cardiac patients—who helped me through my recovery. Most of all, I'd like to thank my wife, Jayne; she was uncomfortable with this project because she didn't want to relive bad memories, but she put that aside and became an editor and collaborator for large parts of this book. It's a better book because she helped, and I thank her for that—and for everything else.

FOREWORD

America's baby boomers, those born between 1945 and 1960, are entering midlife and are beginning to experience the health-related consequences of three or four decades of the American lifestyle. One of these consequences is coronary artery disease, also known as heart disease. For the many who survive a heart attack, the coronary event can mark the beginning of a whole new heart-healthful lifestyle. There is, for them, a second chance, a chance to cheat heart disease of its debilitating grip on their generation.

The first step in rehabilitation is to accept full responsibility for managing your own health. Of course, the road to acceptance of heart disease, or any long-term illness, is not direct. Many deny the seriousness of their illness; some deny even the diagnosis itself.

When denial is no longer possible, bargaining may begin. You ask your physician or nurse, "If I stop eating saturated fat altogether and stop smoking today, will my heart disease go away? Will my heart attack be reversed?" You already know the answers to these questions and the futility of such reasoning. But it takes time to admit it, and, when you do, the "Why me?" anger begins. You will say to yourself, "No one else in my family has a heart problem," "I'm not that much overweight," or "I'm too young to have a heart attack." Your anger is well founded. But, ultimately, there is no one to blame, and so there is no appropriate target for your anger. Your anger will fall at times on those closest to you: your spouse and children. This, of course, adds to your guilt—and your anger.

This sequence of denial, bargaining, anger, and guilt is almost a rite of passage. But, once the ritual is completed, you must accept the reality of the circumstances and address the serious challenge of ministering to your own health. Cardiac rehabilitation, like any self-improvement effort, requires personal commitment. You, the patient, must become the principal agent in the management of your health; no one else can do it for you.

Certainly you may and must recruit others into your health management program—nurses, dietitians, exercise physiologists, physical and occupational therapists, physicians and surgeons, and other heart patients. It's easy to decide whom to recruit and consult regarding medical/surgical strategies, choice of medications, decisions about whether to choose surgical intervention, and so on. Here, you must have physicians. But the larger and more challenging responsibility for developing a heart-healthful lifestyle falls squarely on the patient. This responsibility means, in large part, that you must make major changes in the way you live, reversing many of the health-threatening behaviors that got you into this predicament.

It's up to you. If you are married, I suggest that your spouse become co-director of the rehabilitative effort. He or she is involved in your illness in real and intimate ways. Often the spouse feels cheated in much the same way that the patient does. His or her earning power is compromised and expenses are increased; the spouse feels resentment, anger, and guilt.

Over nearly a decade and a half of working with cardiac patients, I have often been moved by the magnificence of the human spirit when faced with severe challenges. This magnificence is always there, I presume, but it remains latent except during extreme adversity. Heart disease can provide an opportunity to affirm one's personal strength. In a similar way, the spouse can often affirm the highest virtue of his or her own human spirit in the selfless caring for and nurturing of the patient.

As you develop your own heart-healthful lifestyle, perhaps you can inoculate your children against heart disease. You can lead them by your example toward healthful eating behaviors, a nicotine-free life, and an appreciation of the importance and joy of an active life.

Let's get high on health. Jim Castelli did it after his heart attack. I like to think I helped him. Maybe through this book, he can help you to do it, too. Good luck.

James A. Metcalf, Ph.D.
Associate Professor of Health
Sport and Leisure Studies
George Mason University

Exercise Physiologist
Cardiac Rehabilitation
Fairfax Hospital
Fairfax, VA

CONTENTS

I'm Too Young To Have a Heart Attack

1

HEART ATTACK

My heart attack occurred when I was feeling better than I could remember ever feeling in my life. It was June 1985, seven weeks after my thirty-eighth birthday. I had just gone through a strange transition. Three months earlier, I had accidentally discovered that I was addicted to caffeine. I was a Tab™-aholic, with a six-pack-a-day habit. I had a minor medical problem that was aggravated by caffeine, and my doctor had told me to stay off it for a while. I developed a horrible headache and I couldn't put two words together—a bad state for a writer. I was going through caffeine withdrawal. I felt much better once I got detoxed, but there was a bonus as well: I started to lose weight without even trying. Not wanting to look a gift horse in the mouth, I'd started exercising again, working out on a rowing machine. I had lost 25 pounds, getting thin enough to wear baggy pants—the kind with the pleats that, as a kid, I had thought were old-fashioned when my father wore them.

Even though I was feeling good in general, for four or five days before the attack, I felt a little off. Sometimes I just ran out of steam; a few times when I exerted myself outside, running with our Great Pyrennes puppy, Willie, or climbing a hill, I just pulled up short of breath. I had a constricted feeling across my chest that reminded me of the two or three times I'd had asthmatic bronchitis. But because the humidity and pollution levels were intolerable—a typical Washington summer—I assumed that the problem was caused by my allergies. After a few days, I took some pills that had worked the last time I had had a touch of asthmatic bronchitis. This time they did nothing.

The day before the heart attack, I had had a day-long meeting in Alexandria, Virginia. When the meeting was over, I called Jayne from the Pentagon subway stop to tell her which bus I was going to take home. Her boss's wife had just died, and we had to go to a service that evening. We decided that, to save time, I'd take an earlier bus, which had a slightly different route. It would leave me at Rolling Valley Mall, a nearby shopping center, and Jayne would pick me up. I had to run for the bus and was surprised that it bothered me only a little bit. The bus got stuck in traffic on I-395 South and took 45 minutes longer than usual to get to my stop.

When I finally got to Rolling Valley Mall, there was no sign of Jayne. I looked around for a while and when I couldn't find her, I called home. "Where are you?" she screamed into the phone. When a different bus had pulled up at exactly the right time and I hadn't gotten off, she got worried. After waiting awhile, she went back home, thinking I'd missed the first bus and taken the later bus. When I didn't get off that one either, some instinct took over and she did something she'd never done before. She began calling hospital emergency rooms, fearing that I'd had some kind of attack while running for the bus at the Pentagon. That's not nearly as crazy as it sounds. Over the years, Jayne's intuition has been in-credible. I keep asking her if she ever gets visions of horses with numbers on them but, so far, she hasn't.

After the service that evening, we ate at our favorite pizza place. On the way home, we stopped at the Giant supermarket. I bought some over-the-counter asthma medicine, thinking that if I didn't feel better in a few days, I'd see a doctor. Later, Jayne fell asleep holding me and crying.

The next morning, I took a couple of the pills before breakfast. After breakfast, I took Willie out for a walk. I got about two houses up the street, and I couldn't breathe—it was as though my whole chest were clenching up, cutting off the air. I dragged Willie back into the house and began calling up to Jayne. It was only 7:45, and she was still in the bedroom with the door closed. She couldn't hear me.

Matt and Dan, our sons, were sound asleep, enjoying the first days of summer. By now, I was lying on the floor, trying to rest. I knew I couldn't make it up the stairs to get Jayne, so I managed to go downstairs to my office, where I had a separate phone line. I called Jayne on our home phone. As it turned out, she had been about to get into the shower but stopped because Willie was making a com-motion. She went to see why just as the phone rang. When she answered, I said, "You've got to get me to Fam-ily Care." This was a local walk-in "doc-in-the-box" emer-gency center. Even then, I thought it was some nasty form of bronchitis.

I hung up the phone and tried to get comfortable, but no position—sitting, standing or lying down—was even tolerable. The clenched, constricted feeling had been joined by sharp pain in my back and left arm and real nausea. They were all the classic heart attack symptoms that everyone thinks they've had at some time or other, but they all felt qualitatively different—and far worse—than any of the pseudo-symptoms I had ever felt. To make matters worse, Willie was jumping all over me. At first, I thought he was just trying to play, but then I realized that his rescue-dog instincts had taken over and he was trying to "rescue" me. He covered me with this body, licked my face, turned and nipped at my ankles. I realized I was in deep trouble—and that it wasn't bronchitis.

In no more than a minute or two, Jayne was dressed and at the front door yelling, "Let's go," but I couldn't get up off the floor. "Get somebody here," I hollered. "I can't breathe." At least that's what I thought I hollered; Jayne said I never made a sound. She called the 911 emergency number to get the paramedics. The woman who answered first kept asking if I had had an allergic reaction to the pills I had taken, but Jayne told her, "Just get somebody here—my husband is on the floor and he can't breathe." The woman finally said she'd send someone. She asked for our phone number, and we later learned that, following standard procedure, she had cut off our phone line so that no one else could tie it up and she could get back to us if necessary.

In the minute it took for the paramedics to arrive, Jayne asked if my chest hurt and I said something about "crushing" and "heavy." She asked if my left arm hurt, and I said yes. She took my pulse—it was 96 and steady—and felt that my skin was clammy; I looked gray. She thought about the old "I Am Joe's Heart" article in *Reader's Digest* and knew what was happening.

The paramedics came from a fire station exactly one mile away. Willie, still trying to rescue me, wouldn't let the paramedics near me. One of them had to pick him up bodily and put him out in the back yard—no easy feat, because he weighed 65 pounds at six months. They asked me questions about the kind of pain I had and gave me a nitroglycerin tablet to see if it helped; I said it didn't. The crew saw enough to know it was a heart attack, and the leader called in for a special cardiac backup unit. As they put me on a stretcher and carried me out of the house, I thought, "38 years old, fuck it, I ain't going. I'm going to be one of those people who say their heart attack saved their life." I later read that panic is a real risk for heart attack victims; I never panicked, maybe because I was too stupid, but I was vaguely aware that minutes counted, and I felt safe now that I had made it into the medical care system. I was conscious during the ride to Commonwealth Hospital. I kept hearing "Ten minutes till arrival . . . seven minutes . . ." Jayne rode up front and jumped when she heard a paramedic describe my vital signs as "still," but he assured her that that meant steady, not stopped, and said that if my pulse did stop, they had the equipment to get it started again.

I remember being wheeled into the emergency room. When a nurse—Malcolm, roly-poly, wearing glasses and mutton-chop sideburns—said he was going to pull my shoes off, I said, "Take the socks, too, even though I may be sorry for it."

"I'll be sorry?" he asked.

I said, "No, it's just that my feet will get cold." I was aware of activity all around me. Then they sat me up to take a chest X-ray, and I blacked out.

Malcolm had watched me since I came in; his instincts had told him that I was going to go sour, and he stood ready with the paddles that are used to electrically shock the heart. I blacked out because the attack had occurred in the area of the heart that generates electrical activity; it had made my pulse rate soar until it was beating at two hundred to three hundred beats a minute. Because the heart cannot sustain that rate, the doctors had to slow it down. That meant first stopping it, so Malcolm applied the first shock to stop my heart. I now had a flat EKG. At this point, the cardiac care unit had arrived, responding to an "M-set," Commonwealth's equivalent of a "Code Blue." The unit's nurse supervisor, Eileen, took over; another nurse later told me, "Basically, Jim, we jump-started you." The first few times, the heartbeat was not sufficient to keep me alive; it took three more stop-starts—for a total of four flat EKGs, although for only a matter of seconds—before they got an acceptable heart-beat. The thing doctors fear most in such cases is loss of oxygen to the brain for more than four minutes; that results in such serious brain damage that they ask the family if they want the patient resuscitated.

The next thing I remember was incredible pain in my chest, which was being beaten. This was the cardipulmonary resuscitation (CPR) that finally restored me. I couldn't see anything; my glasses were off, and the oxygen mask had slid up between my eyes so that everything was blurred. With each punch, I screamed into the mask, "Holy shit! Oh, my God! Fuck." As consciousness returned more fully, I began calling for Jayne—"Where's my wife? I want my wife!" Than I said, "Can she hear me? I don't want to upset her," as though she weren't upset enough already by now. As it turned out, no one heard what I was yelling; I'm not sure whether this was because I never actually vocalized my thoughts or because the sound was just muffled by the oxygen mask. When I later told one of the nurses about my screaming, she said, "That's all right, we've heard that word in that room before." As I became more coherent, I realized that the tiny room was full. "How many people are in here?" I asked and was told, "Quite a crowd." I think someone later said there were 13 people in the room. They tell me I kept asking what time it was, although I only remember asking about it once. "Ten to nine," someone said; it felt as though an eternity had gone by, and I asked "At night?" No, it was still morning.

While I was oblivious to what was going on, Jayne had the hard job—getting me admitted while she was scared half to death. Someone asked her whether we had insurance, and Jayne kept pointing to the Blue Cross card she had already produced. "No, dear, I mean life insurance." Jayne called a friend, Ellen, who worked ten minutes away and came right over. The emergency room team called in Dr. Robert Herron, a local cardiologist who had just left the hospital after making his rounds. The first thing Jayne was told was that I'd had a massive heart attack; the emergency room doctor—Jayne never got his name—told her I wasn't going to make it. Later, Herron asked if she would allow the use of a controversial experimental drug that had a 30 percent chance of reopening the artery that had been blocked off. The problem was that the drug also had serious possible adverse effects, including possibly triggering arrhythmia or another attack. Jayne asked if my chances were any worse with traditional treatment; when Herron said they weren't, she refused use of the drug. Ellen turned to the internist who had been called in, Dr. Neeraj Bhushan, and said, "If that were your wife in there, would you use it?" He said he wouldn't; he had just attended a seminar on the drug and said it was too controversial. (That drug and other similar ones are now used routinely and safely.)

I woke up in the Coronary Care Unit, hooked up to what seemed like a million machines and with tubes down my nose. Dr. Herron came in to tell me what had happened. I remember hearing something about plaque and the anterior artery. I was pretty dazed, and when he mentioned plaque, I thought that a heart attack was a pretty severe punishment for not flossing my teeth, but I soon figured out that "plaque" was another word for the deposits that had clogged my artery. Remembering that my "posterior" was my rear end, I also figured out that "anterior" meant that the blockage was in the artery in the front of my heart, whatever that meant. Herron said that the attack had done considerable damage; he was sober but reassuring, telling me that the first four hours were particularly crucial and that the first 24 to 48 critical. Jayne later told me that Eileen, the nurse supervisor, sat by my bed and didn't take her eyes off me for the whole first four hours.

When I first saw Jayne, I told her I felt all right and

tried to reassure her. When she first saw me, a bizarre image flashed through her head. She had recently teased me that I was getting stodgy and should start wearing a diamond earring to perk up my image. I had said, "Over my dead body," and for just a second, she seemed to see one. We had left without even waking up Matt and Dan. Jayne said another neighbor, Don, had told them what had happened as he was watching out for them.

My mind was racing. I knew I needed a long rest, so I gave her the names and phone numbers of people who were expecting work from me within the next few weeks to tell them to forget it. Then I had her call George Gallup, with whom I was working on a book, and our editor at Doubleday to extend a January deadline. (A few years before, George had written a book based on interviews with people who had had "near-death experiences." One of the first things I thought after I came to was, "I'll have to tell George I didn't see any long tunnels or bright lights.") At one level, my thinking in having Jayne make the calls was perfectly lucid—I was buying time to recuperate both short-term and long-term. But at another level, it was perfectly ludicrous; I had poor Jayne phoning people who asked, "Did it happen yesterday?" She would have to tell them, "No, an hour ago." She had to cope with everyone else's shock; some cried, some asked questions she couldn't answer, and one person was so upset he practically hung up on her.

My chest was killing me from the CPR—the muscles ached and it was impossible to get comfortable. The worst was an automatic blood pressure cuff that squeezed my arm to take my pressure every two minutes, like a hi-tech Japanese water torture. I was getting nitroglycerin intravenously. When I complained about pain, a nurse asked if I wanted more morphine; I gave her a funny look, and she said, "Don't worry. You won't get addicted with the amount we give you." I joked that between the morphine and the nitroglycerin, I felt like a terrorist—

meet my demands or I'll blow us all up. There was only one time during the whole stay that I was really afraid: I felt a new pain in my chest and, for the first time in the hospital, pain down my left arm. I thought, "This is it, another attack," but it was just fatigue—another dose of morphine took care of it. There was another brief scare when Dr. Bhushan said my blood sugar level was high and he was concerned because sometimes a heart attack can trigger diabetes. It turned out that the reading had been borderline—I had, after all, been getting an intravenous glucose diet—and my blood sugar level never posed a problem again.

The occasion was not without its lighter moments. At one point, an English nurse appeared over me with a urinal and said, "Hello, I'm Bussy. Do you have to go wee-wee? Do you need help putting George in the bottle?" In fact, "George" was hiding, but I managed. Later, another nurse, who had looked over the medical history Jayne had provided, noted that I'd had prostatitis on occasion and asked if it bothered me now. "No," I answered, "it only acts up when I'm under stress." Later, it seemed a pretty funny thing to say. But I thought about it again and realized that stress takes time; what I had undergone was a shock. There was further proof the next morning—Jayne noticed the first gray hairs in my beard. A nurse told her that was not unheard of, either.

Jayne had spent the night at the hospital, getting what little sleep she could in a chair. A nurse sat down and talked to her; she used a plastic model of the heart to show Jayne what had happened to me and why my attack had been so severe. She said that if I had had an attack when I was older, I probably would have had some "collateral circulation"—smaller arteries open up and form a detour around a blockage in a coronary artery to keep blood flowing to the heart. Collateral circulation lessens the severity of an attack; I didn't have any.

Between the shock and the drugs, the days I spent in

the Coronary Care Unit are still pretty much a blur. I didn't put on my glasses for the whole four days and I never even wore a hospital gown. I was tossing enough that I was constantly tangled up with the sheets, and I didn't want to get tangled up in the gown, too. I remember incidents, but, except for a few things that happened on my last day in the unit, it's almost impossible to remember the order in which they happened. I know that Jayne slept at the hospital the first night, and through the middle of the second night. The first night, the doctors were still watching me very closely, and someone said Jayne could go home. She said she wanted to be there to hold me if I were dying; she was told, "They wouldn't let you do that anyway."

Jayne had Ellen call my sister Terri's office; Terri was out, but Ellen told another woman there what had happened and asked her to be there when she called Terri again. After Jayne and Terri talked, Terri got a ride to pick up my father and they went to the house to stay with the kids while Jayne was at the hospital. They came to the hospital later and my father held my hand. It brought me back 15 years to when he had his heart attack and I held his hand as he lay on a hospital stretcher. (My parents and Terri had moved to Virginia in 1981 after my father retired; my mother died of lung cancer in 1983.)

I looked at my watch constantly. About 8:00 Friday morning, I told my nurse, Beth, "Well, it's 24 hours." She smiled and said, "You're all right." I had two visitors that evening. Technically, only the immediate family was allowed, but Jayne said the visitors were her brothers. I'm sure no one believed her, but they let them in. One was Stan Hastey, a good friend and a neighbor in Burke. Jayne had called him at his office, the Baptist Joint Committee on Public Affairs. She was told that he was in Dallas at the Southern Baptist Convention; he later called her from the press room there. Word soon spread among my reporter friends—Dave Anderson from UPI, Helen

Parmley from the *Dallas Morning News* and Bruce Buursma from the *Chicago Tribune* sent telegrams. Through Stan and his boss, James Dunn, they even prayed for me at the Convention meeting.

The other friend was Frank Butler, whom I had met when he worked in the social justice office at the United States Catholic Conference (USCC) and I worked at National Catholic News Service, part of the USCC. I later joked that Frank had suddenly become the national information clearinghouse on the status of Jim Castelli, passing information along to other friends and colleagues. He had heard in a roundabout way: Jayne had called Tony Podesta at People for the American Way (PFAW), where I was consulting; Melanne Verveer, PFAW's legislative director, who used to work at the USCC, called her friends at USCC to tell them what had happened; a secretary in the USCC office then called Frank. Frank told me that the U.S. Catholic bishops, who were holding a semiannual meeting in Collegeville, Minnesota, had offered special prayers for me. I figured that with the Southern Baptists and Catholics praying for me the same week, I ought to be in good shape. It was a boost seeing friends, and Stan was a big help to Jayne, talking with her for about two hours. Jayne fell asleep in a chair in the waiting room, and when she woke up, she felt better because Stan was still sitting there. Jayne was also touched by the fact that her boss, Dr. Heenan, had come to the hospital to see us the evening of the day he buried his wife.

I felt progressively better each day, particularly as first one machine or tube and then another was removed. The automatic blood pressure cuff was cut back to every 15 minutes and eventually every half hour, so I could rest a bit more. I had my first meal Friday night, and hospital food never tasted so good. Jayne came in one day with a Polaroid camera; Dan didn't believe I was still alive, so she had to bring him a picture. I smiled and waved, grateful that at this point I only had the oxygen tube in my nose. (Earlier, I was aware of another tube down my nose; it didn't bother me until they took it out and I realized how far down it had gone.)

On Sunday, three of the paramedics who had brought me to the emergency room stopped by to say hello and see how I was doing. I was glad to see them, and Dr. Herron later said it was important for them to stop by like that because they often don't know what happens to the people they bring in, and they need to see their successes. It was also good to hear that I was a "success."

Sunday was Father's Day, and Jayne brought Matt and Dan by for the first time. They brought my Father's Day presents, including a mug with a cow on it that said— what else?—"De Calf." I also got a new watch with laser images instead of hands; in all the confusion, we lost the instructions, and I never did figure out how to set it.

In many ways, our kids were clones of Jayne and me. Both had brown hair and large brown eyes. Dan had Jayne's high, round, adorable cheeks. Also, like Jayne, he wore his feelings close to the surface—he always spoke up, and if he had a problem, he talked about it. Matt was more like me, quiet and close-mouthed about feelings.

Matt was fine while he was with me, but he cried when he got out in the hall. Dan was very tentative at first; I had to tell him it was all right to hug me hard. I told him several times that I was all right. He didn't seem to believe me at first, but I must have finally said it in a way that convinced him, because he finally asked, "You are OK?" When I said I was, he went bouncing out of the room and told Jayne, "Dad's all right. He told me."

Sunday was my fourth day in the hospital. A nurse told me I was being moved into the Progressive Care Unit that evening to get ready to go home in about a week. The difference between making the move on Sunday night and making it on Monday morning was significant. A Sunday move was the best Father's Day present of all—it meant I was going to live. Two nurses wheeled me across the hall to the new unit; Jayne, my father, Stan, Frank, and Dr. Heenan were in the hall, and they all applauded as I rode by.

2

PROGRESSIVE CARE UNIT

"You're not weak because you had a heart attack. You're weak because you've just spent four days in bed."

That was the first thing I heard after being moved into the Progressive Care Unit. It came from a nurse and was a refrain I heard often in my first few days there. It captured the new philosophy of cardiac care—the sooner people get up and around, the better off they'll be. When my father had a heart attack in 1970, the doctors kept him in the hospital for six weeks. That marked progress. When President Eisenhower had a mild heart attack in the '50s, he was in the hospital for seven weeks. "In those days," one of my nurses said, "the cure killed you."

The move from the Coronary Care Unit to the Progressive Care Unit marked more than a shift in medical treatment. It also marked a shift in attitude and focus. First, I was on considerably less medication and, although I was still exhausted, I could stay awake and, therefore, coherent, for longer periods of time. The shock hadn't completely worn off. But I now had some assurance that I was, in fact, going to live. This was the time to begin thinking about what that meant. The next week would be a period of education and re-education. I had to find out just what had happened to me—and how to make sure that it didn't happen again.

This new phase began symbolically on Monday morning when I had my first shave since Wednesday. I wear a beard, but I still shave below it, and by Monday my neck was pretty scratchy. They wouldn't let me shave myself yet, but Bussy did a pretty good job.

I also began to get a sense of my context. I thought that, at 38, I was too young to have a heart attack. But my nurses told me that wasn't necessarily the case anymore—the average age of those in the Progressive Care Unit, all men, was 42. There were two reasons for that, they said. First, men were having heart attacks at an earlier age. Second, the survival rate was highest among younger men because they had the strength to fight back. I'd never had so many people tell me how young and strong I was before, even though I didn't feel like either.

I started to ask myself the universal question after a catastrophe, "Why me?" I also asked "How me?" My nurses told me there are three major risk factors for a heart attack—smoking, high blood pressure, and high cholesterol. I didn't have any of them. I was comparatively young, and I'd played by the rules reasonably well—this shouldn't have happened. But I hadn't been perfect. I was overweight; I couldn't even say I was out of shape because that would imply that I had ever been in shape, and I hadn't, except for the past few months. I did eat an occasional ham and egg muffin and a bacon cheeseburger. But I'd been given something of a clean bill of health two and a half years before after a freak episode.

It was a cold day in February, and I began having severe pains in my chest and down my left arm. I thought, of course, that I was too young to be having a heart attack, but the symptoms were classic. As it happened, it was the day that Karen Carpenter died at 32 of "heart failure." At least, the doctors called it that before they knew she was an anorexic, so a heart attack for me seemed possible. We lived in Alexandria, Virginia, at the time, and I went to the emergency room at Alexandria Hospital. It turned out I had a bad flu that mimicked many heart attack symptoms. By a month later, almost everyone I knew had had it, and people were calling it "the heart attack flu." I had just been one of the first to get it. (I'm often among the first to get a new bug. Sometimes I think I should open a flu consulting service—"This is how you'll know you have it, and this is what it feels like on the second day . . .")

The cardiologist the hospital called in said my triglycerides—blood fats—were a little high, but he saw no other problems. He had me come in for a treadmill stress test, which knocked me out. He said, "You'd be in good shape if you were 65." Then he told me to exercise and lose weight, but there was no sign of imminent danger and I wasn't told to do anything other than get ordinary checkups.

What I did have going against me, apparently, was genetics. My father was 51 when he had his heart attack; his sister, Ida, had died of a heart attack at 42; and my mother's brother, Reuben, had died of one at 52. I should have taken all that a lot more seriously.

But as I thought about it, I realized I did have some genetic factors in my favor. My father was still alive and well; he had been the second youngest of ten children, and his older brothers and sisters were doing well. I thought back to the day my mother died two years earlier. She had developed lung cancer after 50 years of a two-pack-a-day smoking habit—her smoking had turned my sister and me off to cigarettes long ago. When she was in the terminal stages, her doctor called my father at about five in the morning to ask permission not to resuscitate, and he gave it; she was unconscious and they expected her to go at any minute. We all went to the hospital. She held out until about eight that night; her heart kept beating even when her blood pressure was almost gone. I remember thinking, "Her heart was strong after all." Then—the most obvious genetic factor in my favor—I was still here. I had survived what I heard described, more times than I cared to, as a "massive" attack. That had to count for something.

Recovery would take some fighting, but I realized I'd been fighting for so long I didn't even recognize it. I had had serious vision problems ever since birth; I was extremely nearsighted, with severe astigmatism and a nystagmus in my right eye—it tended to drift because I didn't have full control of the muscles there. I thought back to the year I graduated from college, 1969. I knew all along that there was no question that my classification for the draft would be 4-F because of my eyes, but as my student deferment ran out, I had to get the classification done officially. I got a letter from my eye doctor saying that I was legally blind—my corrected vision was 20-400 in my right eye and 20-200 in my "good" eye. After I got the paperwork done, I received a surprise visit from a representative of the New York State Commission for the Blind. I remember clearly two things he said. The first was, "Gee, if we knew about you earlier, we'd have paid all your college tuition and bought you a new typewriter." The second was how surprised he was at what I had already done. He said, "I see people with your vision sitting in a corner stringing beads for a living."

That was exactly what my parents had worked hard to avoid, and I grew up knowing I had to make certain adjustments—like walking up to the front of the room to copy things off the blackboard at school—but trying to be as normal as possible. The second time I got hit in the head with a baseball, I stopped playing hardball—my friends and I switched to whiffle ball—but I was out there

trying. One doctor told me my vision would actually improve as I got older, because the natural tendency is to
get farsighted as you age. That had been the case; at one
point, with contact lenses, the vision in my left eye was 20-
70, good enough to get a driver's license for daytime
only. But after I had spent about a thousand dollars on
driving lessons, I realized that even though my distance
vision was better, I still couldn't control my gaze enough
to drive safely. You drive where you look, and I couldn't
shake a tendency to look at cars coming toward me, a condition that made a head-on collision inevitable. I gave up
the contacts and dreams of driving; you have to know
when to say no. It was funny, though—I was really good
at parking because that's something you do up close. It's
just like reading; people always assume that because I
hold things close when I read I'm having a problem. The
fact is, I can't read at a distance, but within my range, I
read as well as anyone and better than most. So as I
thought about the new fight ahead, I felt better knowing
I'd had some experience fighting the odds; I didn't, after
all, make my living stringing beads.

As these thoughts were running through my head, I
gained a roommate, Lou, whose story made my experience look like a picnic. The doctors had had to give me
electroshock and CPR four times before they got a stable
heartbeat. They did it to him 15 times over a period of an
hour and a half. And this was his second heart attack.
Now that's strong. The nurses called us "the miracle
boys."

Lou's grandchildren came to visit and brought him a
stuffed whale. Jayne thought it was a good idea and came
back with a stuffed Garfield doll. We have a large, orange
cat named Garfield, so the doll was a reminder of home as
well as something to hold onto. That night, while Lou
and I were sleeping with our stuffed animals, I heard one
nurse say, "They've both got one," and another say, "The
guy in the next room has one, too."

Jayne also brought me the trappings of normalcy: my reading glasses, a mystery—*Siskiyou* by Richard Hoyt— and a portable radio. When I turned on the country station I listen to, the first thing I heard was Steve Wariner singing "Heart Trouble."

It was time to find out just what my own "heart trouble" was. That wasn't as easy as it might seem. My doctors explained that without knowing what my heart looked like the day before my attack, they couldn't say exactly what had happened. The most likely explanation was a blockage in the anterior artery. But, they said, they didn't know whether that was a 99 percent blockage that went to 100 percent, or a 70 percent blockage—not considered serious—that hemorrhaged and caused a clot. Another possibility was that the artery had gone into spasm, choking off the flow of blood to the heart.

I also read about the collateral circulation the nurse had explained to Jayne. If my attack had come ten years later, I probably would have developed some collateral circulation, which would have made the heart attack less severe. But at the same time, in ten years I might not be as strong as I was today and it might be harder to survive or recover.

As I studied all this, I realized that if I still couldn't answer the "Why?" of my heart attack, I could make a good guess at the "How?" It seemed most likely to me that I'd had a coronary artery blockage that had reached 100 percent. The couple of times I'd been short of breath after very little exertion the week before my attack must have signaled the final narrowing of the artery.

Between adjusting to being out of the Coronary Care Unit and studying my heart books, I was exhausted. That evening, though, I learned about two hospital rituals that made me feel a little better. The first was my bedtime snack—we all got milk (skim) and cookies. It strikes me now that the hospital knew that "Warm cookies and cold milk are good for you" before Robert Fulghum elevated the notion to folk wisdom. I think the hospital's reasoning was that we'd sleep better with something in our stomachs. I knew there was a good reason I always nibbled at bedtime.

The second ritual was the nightly backrub. After all the CPR I had received, my chest hurt, deep in the muscles and bones. A backrub was medicinal. It relaxed the muscles all through the back and chest. They told me to just ring the nurse's button if I needed a backrub. It was hard not to take advantage.

Tuesday began with another adventure—my first shampoo in almost a week. Grooming took a back seat, but my head itched, and it was difficult to scratch it. Arm motion is the most tiring for the heart, and I had to work my way up to it. So we pulled a chair over in front of the bathroom sink, and Bussy washed my hair. She half drowned me, but we laughed a lot.

It sounds funny to talk about laughing less than a week after a massive heart attack, but it was quite natural. I was surprisingly upbeat. A certain exhilaration sets in. It must be something like the feeling people say they get when they get shot at—and missed. The hospital stay was something of an oasis—everybody laughed, my family and friends came to visit and brought me presents, we didn't worry about whether the mortgage and car payment got mailed on time, and there was milk and cookies at bedtime and those backrubs on demand.

It wasn't completely fun, though. The strain was showing on Jayne, who had to handle things at home, reassure Matt and Dan, run errands, and make a million trips to the hospital. And the exhilaration was mixed with apprehension; we still didn't know just what I was facing, and it would be weeks before we would.

One of the hardest things on Jayne was answering the phone and dealing with the same questions about me over and over. She said, "It was like being stuck in a time warp. You were recovering, and I was still reliving the heart attack every time someone who hadn't heard what happened wanted to know. And of course they didn't ask you because they didn't want to upset you by making you relive it. I guess it wasn't supposed to upset me to keep retelling it. No one meant any harm, but it was very hard."

I was upset when they put me on a new medication. I knew I was taking some pills, but I really wasn't sure what they were at this point. On Tuesday, Bussy told Dr. Herron that I seemed to be breathing a little harder than I should be. He decided to put me on Lanoxin, a brand of digitalis, an old heart-strengthening drug. It comes from the foxglove plant; Bussy said she used to work for a doctor who used to say, "Time for a touch of the old foxglove." The medication is just a little white pill, but before you take that, you get a large dose through a process called "digitalizing"—an injection through the back of the hand. It hurts. After I got "digitalized," a nurse named Nancy picked up on the fact that I felt a little down. She told me that getting the digitalis did not mark a "setback"; most heart patients take it in some form.

It seemed, at least, that my heart attack might help some of my friends. It was amazing how many of them vowed to quit smoking, lose weight, and get back to their exercise programs.

I was supposed to begin physical therapy, but, in my newfound freedom, I ate a big lunch—even with hospital food. When the therapist, a German woman named Lily, came by after lunch, I was too stuffed and tired to move. Therapy would begin tomorrow.

Tuesday's education consisted of a film about a procedure I could look forward to—the angiogram, or cardiac catheterization. This involved a doctor's inserting a catheter into the femoral artery in the groin on the right side and injecting a dye that would show up on film, revealing what was going on inside my heart and arteries. This would show the extent of the damage to the heart and the size and location of any blockages in the arteries.

If there were blockages of more than 70 percent, I would probably have to have surgery. There were two possibilities. The most common was a coronary bypass, in which the doctors build a new artery around the blockages with a vein removed from the leg. A newer procedure was balloon angioplasty, in which the doctors insert a catheter, as used in an angiogram, with a balloon on the end. The balloon is then inflated inside the artery to flatten out the blockage. The size and position of the blockage usually determine which procedure is used. If the angiogram showed no significant blockages, I'd be treated with diet, exercise, and medication.

I certainly hoped there were no more blockages. I figured I could probably handle the angioplasty if it came to it, but I dreaded the prospect of having my chest cut open and a bypass done. Actually, I think I dreaded the anticipation and looking forward to surgery about as much. My heart attack had come suddenly, and I was past it and starting to recover practically before I knew what hit me. Surgery would be different; I'd have days and probably weeks to worry about it. But I knew that if I had to do it, I had to do it. Sometimes there aren't a lot of options.

I began Wednesday by getting a new roommate. They moved Lou to another hospital to do his angiogram. (He had severe pain in his chest from the repeated CPR, but he also had temporary short-term memory loss from his experience; he kept asking why his chest hurt. One of the nurses joked, "If he asks one more time, I'm going to hit him again.")

My new roommate was an older man named Denny who had just had a pacemaker installed. After it was in, his doctors found that they had to adjust it because it was kicking in sooner than it was needed, at something like 55 beats per minute instead of 70. That sounded frightening—how do you adjust a pacemaker? Well, his doctor came in the next night with a computer keyboard and something that looked like a hairdryer. He hit a few keys and—Voila!—the pacemaker was adjusted.

In the afternoon, I turned to my "homework" again. I now had, in addition to the booklets the hospital gave me, several books that Jayne had found. She had combed area bookstores looking for everything that might help. She found some cookbooks (including the *The American Heart Association Cookbook*) and a good book on stress. What she couldn't find, because it apparently didn't exist, was a book that would tell me what it would be like and feel like for me from here on in. That's when I decided to write exactly that book. That was the personal side of it. I also had a professional angle. The oldest rule in writing is to write about what you know, and I now knew about a whole new subject, up close and personal. I remember thinking, "If Bob Greene can get a book by keeping a diary after his wife had a baby, I can get a book out of this." Jayne brought me a pen and notebook, and I began making cryptic notes to myself. Some were a little too cryptic—I either can't read them today or have no idea what they mean.

That day I read a little about the relationship between stress and heart disease and the role of exercise, which includes sex. I read *Stress, Diet and Your Heart* by Dr. Dean Ornish, and I learned that stress increases heart rate, blood pressure, breathing rate, and muscle tension. It also produces chemical changes that make artery spasms and platelet clumping more likely and, in addition, raises the level of cholesterol in the blood. I thought, "Bingo," and bells went off in my head; I was used to living in constant stress, and I could easily see how it had helped get me where I was.

One way to deal with stress is exercise, and all the materials the hospital gave me emphasized the importance of exercise. At one level, people who exercise have a lower rate of heart attack than people who don't. At another level, exercise is the best way to get the heart in shape after an attack. The pamphlets all said the proper exercise was cardiovascular—walking, running, jogging, cycling, swimming. The choice was easy for me. I'd never really learned how to swim. I had to pass a swimming test to pass gym class in order to graduate from high school; if it weren't for a tolerant gym teacher who accepted a good faith effort, I'd still be in high school. I'd tried a cycling machine, but a couple of years ago I'd had some minor surgery that now made sitting on a bicycle seat extremely painful. But I could walk, and I'd always been a walker. My father was famous for walking with long strides, and the rest of us could never keep up with him. I figured if I had his heart, it would help balance things off if I had his legs, too. The walking program the hospital recommended would begin as soon as I got home. The goal of the program was to have me walk a mile in 15 minutes.

The most popular pamphlet the hospital gave me—the one I showed to everyone who came to visit—is called "The Sensuous Heart." On the cover, it has a cartoon of a smiling heart carrying flowers. The gist of the pamphlet is that sex after a heart attack is all right—and good. A major problem is that many heart attack victims, who were mostly men, anyway, are afraid that sex will cause another attack and probably kill them. Except for the most unusual cases, this is not true. The booklet offers a simple comparison—if you can climb two flights of stairs without being short of breath, you can have sex safely.

Reading about stress made me stop and think. I was determined to relax and enjoy life more. But I didn't really know what that meant on a day-to-day basis. I practically had to interview myself—what did I like to do? First, I realized the obvious—I really did enjoy being with my family. One thing that had always kept Jayne and me together was our sense of humor. We could always find something to laugh about, even in the worst of times. I joked that the fourth slice of pizza I'd had the night before my attack had brought my arteries to critical mass.

Jayne countered that my attack was a delayed reaction to spending almost five hours at an avant-garde production of *The Count of Monte Cristo* at the Kennedy Center the week before.

I enjoyed talking with Matt and Dan; they had inherited the family sense of humor and were genuinely interesting kids. I had another revelation of the obvious. Jayne always kidded me that whenever we went shopping, no matter where we were, I always ended up looking at books and records. (When we went to London three months earlier, I had dragged back a half dozen cassettes and what felt like a ton of books.) Well, I *liked* books and records; now I'd buy them without guilt as part of my new stress-reduction plan.

I had some more clinical discussions with several nurses during the day on the theme of "denial." I think I was starting to feel guilty for having a heart attack. I should have taken better care of myself. But they told me my feelings were only natural—everyone indulges in some form of denial. I felt I was immune because of my age. One nurse said she smoked even though she knew better. Another said she knew she was overweight and had a very stressful job, but felt "safe" because she didn't smoke. Another said she was overweight and didn't eat right, but felt "safe" because she had not yet gone through menopause. "My hormones are protecting me," she said.

If Wednesday offered a bit of a lull, Thursday was a busy, busy day. It began on a happy note. When I woke up early in the morning, I noticed that "George" was wide awake, too, almost one week to the minute after my heart attack. That was reassuring. I looked at my watch, rolled over, opened my notebook, took a pen, and wrote down "4:54 A.M." I added a short note so I'd remember why I wrote the time down.

About an hour later, I was in the bathroom when I heard a banging on the door and a nurse's voice yelling,

"Are you all right?" I told her that I was. When I came out, I discovered the reason for her panic. Since coming into this unit, I had worn a portable heart monitor about the size of a transistor radio. It sent signals out to a console, where nurses could monitor all the patients in the unit on TV-like screens. I had suddenly disappeared from the screen. The nurse replaced the battery in my monitor, and I reappeared. She left laughing, "Another life saved."

I had another "adventure" in the bathroom that day— the doctors let me take my first shower in a week. Physically, it felt fabulous. I let the warm water run over me, down my aching chest and sore back, as long as I could. Psychologically, it felt even better. There really is something to the symbolism of water as a sign of rebirth. Each time I did something "normal" by myself, I felt more optimistic about recovering. I felt even more optimistic that afternoon during my physical therapy when I was able to walk down the hall on my own.

After my walk, I had to go in for a procedure known as an echocardiogram, essentially a sonogram of the heart. Short of an angiogram, this would give my doctors important information about how well my heart was functioning and whether the clot had cleared up. I lay down on a table and a technician took something that looked like a microphone, pressed it down on my diaphragm, and said, "Take a deep breath." I don't know where she expected me to get it from—I couldn't expand my diaphragm with her leaning on it—but I managed. I had to wait until the next day for the results.

My busy day continued; after the echocardiogram, the hospital dietitian came in to talk to me about my new low-fat, low-cholesterol, low-sodium diet. Some parts of it were easier to understand than others, and some parts of it would be easier to swallow than others.

The American Heart Association recommends eating no more than 300 milligrams of cholesterol a day and eating no more than 30 percent of calories from fat. There were some obvious foods to avoid. First, one egg contained 213 milligrams of cholesterol, over two thirds of a whole day's supply. They recommended no more than three egg yolks a week, but I figured that would be easy. I'd just cut out eggs altogether. Whole milk, cream, butter, and ice cream were also high in cholesterol and fats. Fruits and vegetables were generally fine; olives and tropical oils (coconut and palm) were definite no-nos. On the bright side, I was supposed to increase my intake of complex carbohydrates—breads, rice, pasta, potatoes—which were among my favorite foods.

I was supposed to have red meat no more than three times a week, and then only lean cuts. (The leanness wouldn't be a problem; the last few years I'd noticed that a prime rib didn't hold the same appeal it used to.) I was supposed to eat more fish and poultry than red meat, but I'd have to stick to three-ounce servings of all of them.

The question of fats gets complicated because there are so many different kinds—some good, some bad. The worst are saturated fats, which is anything that hardens at room temperature, such as animal fat or the fat in diary products. Saturated fat raises cholesterol levels. Hydrogenated fats—fats and oils changed from their natural liquid form into solid form such as shortening or margarine—also raise cholesterol levels. Polyunsaturated fats lower cholesterol levels. These include safflower oil, sunflower oil, corn oil, soybean oil, and cottonseed oil. Monounsaturated fats such as olive oil and canola oil are better than saturated and hydrogenated oil, and they may be as good as polyunsaturated oils in lowering cholesterol levels.

Keeping my salt level down proved no problem; I was supposed to have no more than three or four grams of salt in a day, and I normally ate less than half that.

What I liked best about my new diet was its moderation, and that was the whole point. The hospital nutritionist said, "Better a moderate diet that you stick to than a rigid one that you don't." Dr. Herron said, "Does this mean you can never have another cheeseburger? No. If you want a cheeseburger, eat it, enjoy it. Just keep track of it so that over a week, your cholesterol and fat average out to what they should be." Never say "Never," because as soon as someone says you can never eat something again, that's all you think about. I later heard another nutritionist say that even though liver was extremely high in cholesterol—372 milligrams in three ounces—it was all right to have it four times a year. Now, that's about three times a year more than I want it, but every once in a while, I get a yen for liver and onions. The first time I met George Gallup, Jr., in 1981, we formed an instant bond when we both ordered liver and onions for lunch and complained that our wives never made it for us. As a matter of fact, I haven't had liver since my heart attack, but when I pass it over on the menu, it's nice to know I could have it if I really wanted it.

If Thursday was a busy day for me, it was a really bad day for Jayne. She was still stunned and concerned about our future, and she had all of the logistical responsibilities for the family. She was really pushed to the edge by the usual household disasters—two of the three toilets in the house overflowed and she had to get a plumber, and then Willie somehow got hold of a full milk carton and ran around the kitchen biting into it and spraying milk all over. On top of all that, someone broke into our neighbors' car and stole their radio, and the police came to the door asking questions. Jayne still wasn't sleeping—she kept expecting the hospital to call with bad news. When she was at the hospital, she kept running into older women in the cardiac unit who asked her if she were there to visit her father; they looked shocked when she said, "No, my husband." Lou's wife had told her, "You think it gets better when they come home, but it doesn't. It gets worse."

So it's no surprise Jayne was ready to kill me when she came to the hospital after dinner and found me arguing politics with Denny. It was perfectly normal to me. Denny was lively and opinionated, and we just started talking. Before Jayne could strangle me, Tom, a nurse, assured her that we were OK—"I've been taking their blood pressure." And, in fact, he had been doing just that, going back and forth, taking our blood pressure, and laughing, as we got more and more into our debate. Instant stress test—that must have been some scene.

We got news about some other stress reduction. Frank Butler was looking for a way to help out when I went home. He knew that the National Council of Catholic Women had developed a "Respite" program in some areas—a group of volunteers would give some relief to people who were caring for a sick or elderly relative. He asked a friend at the Council if there were such a program in our area. There wasn't, but the friend had an idea—why not just organize our own "Respite"? He volunteered and found three other friends to come by the next week to stay with me for part of the day. That way, Jayne could run errands and just get some time to herself. It sounded like a great idea.

Late Thursday night, I had trouble sleeping. Denny was snoring. I walked down the hall and had a cup of coffee (decaf, with skim milk) with a couple of the nurses and just chatted. This was something else that felt normal.

But there was a flip side to all this "normalcy." It felt good to shower, walk, argue, joke. But I was starting to get antsy. The exhilaration I had felt on Monday was now mixed heavily with apprehension. Was I really going to recover fully, or was I going to be one of those people left out when the books talk about "most" people recovering? I wouldn't know until I got home. In a real sense, today wasn't the first day of the rest of my life. The first day of the rest of my life would be the day I went home.

Friday was the day I was supposed to find out when I was going home; I was hoping for Saturday. I began the day cranky. The nurses couldn't find the results of my cholesterol check, and I went on strike. I wasn't going to eat anything until they did another one. They finally found it, but they told me cholesterol levels right after a heart attack are all but meaningless, anyway. But I figured it was important to make my point.

I felt considerably better when I got the results of my echocardiogram. Dr. Marder, Dr. Herron's partner, said the damage to my heart was less extensive than they had feared. He also said the clot formed by the attack was thinner than before and was dissolving nicely. Everything else looked OK—or as OK as it could, given the circumstances.

What did all that mean for my future? First, it meant I might be able to be treated with just diet and medication, and I might not need angioplasty or a bypass. Second, it meant that my prognosis looked better than it did before they had these results. Overall, I had a lot to be thankful for. Marder said I had been "a half hour away from being a medical statistic." Well, I *was* a medical statistic, one of the 1.5 million people who has a heart attack each year. What he meant was, I was a half-hour away from being a different statistic—one of the half million who die from one.

I felt even better after I did my final physical therapy. I had to go up two flights of stairs at a fairly brisk pace, and I made it with no problem. I figured it was no coincidence that it was two flights of stairs.

Jayne felt better when she got the day's good news. When she came to visit in the afternoon, they let me go with her for a walk through the hospital. We even went out into a courtyard to sit and talk. It was my first time outdoors in more than a week. Like the first shower, the first fresh air felt like a rebirth.

I woke up Saturday morning ready to go home. While

I was waiting to get the OK, I took another walk through the halls and went to get the day's *Washington Post*. I was really daring—I walked outside the range where my portable monitor could be picked up on the console. Reading the paper was funny. I was by nature and profession a news junkie, but I couldn't relate at all to follow-up stories about events that had happened while I was in the Coronary Care Unit.

After I got back to my room and read the paper, I took a shower. I rebelled again. I wasn't going to put on my pajamas. Jayne had brought me clothes—white pleated slacks and a new green checked shirt—and I got dressed and ready to go. Finally, Dr. Herron came in, checked me over, and told me I could go home. (He also told me Lou's angiogram had looked good and he didn't need surgery.) Normally, you must take a short treadmill stress test before the hospital releases you, but, because it was Saturday, they weren't able to do it. They gave me a break and said I could go home anyway; I had passed the stairs test all right. I just had to go to Dr. Bhushan's office next week for the stress test.

Before I left, a nurse drilled me on my medication: Lanoxin, once a day. Procardia, to keep the blood vessels open and blood flowing easily, four times a day; Persantine, to prevent blood clots, three times a day. And an aspirin a day, also to prevent clotting. I could take my pills a half hour early or late. If I forgot a pill, I should take it as soon as I remembered it and not change the rest of my schedule. She also gave me a reduced-size copy of my final EKG to carry in my wallet. That way, if I ever needed an EKG done somewhere else, the doctors would know what damage already existed.

Jayne came for me and, as we were leaving, I put on a new white summer hat I liked. I stopped by the emergency room to thank the crew there, but no one who had worked on me was there because the weekend staff was on. I gave the people who were there my name and said I wanted to leave a message for the crew that had worked on me; I tipped my hat to them. Then, Jayne and I got in the car to go home and start the first day of the rest of my life.

3

COMING HOME

We left the hospital and got into our car, a silver 1981 Ford Escort. The car had cost us a fortune in repairs in the past year but, even so, I was glad to see it.

Within a few minutes, I was home. We had joked that I'd have to spend the first five minutes being greeted by Willie, and that's exactly what I had to do. I just sat down in our front hall and played with him until he settled down. After seeing Matt and Dan and settling in for a few minutes, I walked two houses down to thank Ellen for all the help she'd been to Jayne.

I was restless already. I didn't know what to do with myself, and Jayne wasn't sure what to do with me, either.

There's no other way to say it: the next month was a really bad time. As I look at my "diary" today, I see a number of references that simply say "depressed" (me) or "J[ayne] upset again." There was too much to deal with and not enough help in dealing with it.

First of all, we still didn't know exactly what shape my heart was in, and we wouldn't for about a month, when I would have my angiogram. Second, coming home was a lot like being thrown out of the nest; we had a lot yet to learn and a lot of changes yet to make, but we were flying alone.

I was looking forward—that's putting it mildly—to being able to go to NOVACAT, the cardiac rehabilitation program I'd been told about that was run by the Fairfax Hospital System and George Mason University. But, at the time, a heart patient had to take a full stress test about eight weeks after an attack before being able to join the program. A short time later, NOVACAT began a program for people right out of the hospital; I'd have given almost anything for that kind of help.

At the same time, I was worried about Jayne. One of my biggest complaints about this period is that I couldn't seem to get anyone to take her situation seriously. The only advice that we ever got was "It takes time," which, though true, was totally useless. I remember telling Matt once that maturity isn't like pubic hair: it doesn't just appear one morning; you have to earn it one day at a time. It's the same thing with "time healing"—you still have to go through time one day at a time.

My friend Shannon gave me Norman Cousins's book, *Anatomy of an Illness*, and I spent a lot of time my first few days at home reading it. Cousins wrote about his own experience with a near-fatal disease and the healing power of humor. He believes he virtually laughed himself back to health and makes a strong case that positive thinking leads to good health.

Jayne and I actually had our first post-heart attack fight over that book and my telling everyone how I'd thought "I'm not going" when I'd realized I was having a heart attack. I couldn't understand why she wasn't happy that I had a good attitude. Then she told me why. She was afraid I'd think just having positive thoughts would be enough to protect me and that I'd end up having another attack. The most positive attitude in the world didn't help me while I was unconscious and the cardiac emergency team was working on me. Her point was well taken. I assured her that I knew that the power of positive thinking only went so far.

There was more tension that day. I was impatient with the kids at dinner. When Matt complained that he didn't like the skim milk, I freaked and yelled something stupid like, "That's what's keeping me alive!" I apologized and we worked out the obvious compromise—we'd buy skim milk for me and two percent for the kids.

Jayne said that night that I looked like myself, but I was somehow different. Looking back, I realize that, in order to heal, I had pulled into myself. Jayne felt that as withdrawal, as a pulling away from her and the boys. I reacted to her feelings and drew myself in even more, creating a vicious circle that stayed with us for quite a while. (There was one way in which I didn't look like myself. Just as I had sprouted new gray hair in my beard, I had sprouted a new mole on my back. Jayne noticed it and said she'd keep an eye on it to see if it were growing.)

But there were good days, too, and Monday, the twenty-fourth, was one of them. For one thing, I had started my walking program that day. I was supposed to walk a quarter of a mile in about five minutes. Jayne used the car odometer to find that it was one-tenth of a mile from our house to the entrance of the development. We figured out that by walking to the entrance, coming back to the house, and walking to the corner and back, I'd cover a quarter of a mile.

I was supposed to check my pulse before I walked, as soon as I stopped, and after five minutes. It was 84 beats per minute when I started, went up to 108, and was back to 84 five minutes after I finished walking. That was a good showing. My pulse increased with moderate exercise—as it should—but came back to normal quickly after I stopped. That meant my heart could handle the job; it wasn't overwhelmed by the exertion.

Frank started our "respite" program that day and came by while Jayne went to the mall and the grocery store. I visited with Frank and talked on the phone with David Kusnet and Nancy Stella from People for the American Way. I wasn't working; I was just staying in touch.

My walking went well again on Tuesday. My pulse started at 84, went to 102, and fell back to 84 after five minutes. Mary Esslinger, a friend from National Catholic News Service, was my respite-of-the-day person. But I spent too much time visiting, and this made me very tired.

I was also spending too much time trying to write thank-you notes to everyone who had sent flowers or a card. I got halfway through and wore myself out. I got the nicest note from Gene Kennedy, a psychologist and author. I had only met him briefly a few times, but we knew a lot of the same people, wrote for some of the same publications, and read each other's stuff, so it seemed as if we knew each other better than we did. Gene said it was too bad people had to wait until something like this to hear how much people cared about them. And he gave me some good advice—to take care of myself. He told me not to spend any time writing thank-you notes, including one to him. He was absolutely right; I put my stationery aside and left the thank-yous alone.

Although I never finished my thank-you notes, I did keep a couple of lists in my head. When you go through a crisis like this, there are always surprises in the way other people respond. Some people you expect to come through, and they do. Others you might not have thought of come through and outdo themselves. You never forget either of those groups. Then there's another group of people—the ones you expect to come through, and they don't, they just disappear. I'm lucky that, for me, this was a very small group. I'd be lying, though, if I said I wouldn't remember their names until the day I die. On a practical level, you can't afford to take the time and energy to be overly profusive in your thanks or to be angry at anyone; you need to take care of yourself. People who help help because they want to, not because they're looking for gold stars. And people who disappear aren't worth the energy.

On Wednesday, I was tired and didn't spend much time with John Carr, that day's respite recruit. I had a good deal of chest pain. I was confused, because I couldn't sort out my chest pains—what was from the CPR damage and what was angina? Put another way, did I need to take a nitroglycerin pill or not? Sometimes I did, sometimes I didn't. Sometimes it seemed to help, sometimes it didn't.

Jayne was in bad shape that day. When we talked, she let out what she was feeling—that I was going to die and leave her alone, if not today, in a few years. I did my best to reassure her that I wouldn't. It helped a little. I knew I had to reassure her, but I didn't know how. Looking back, I wonder how the hell I was supposed to.

The day became a little eerie. I went down to my office for the first time since I had come home and played back my answering machine. There were old messages from my friends Al Menendez and Chuck Bergstrom. They had been trying to reach Jayne after first hearing about my attack. The tremors in their voices told me that the word about me on the grapevine wasn't good.

But the day actually ended on a better note. Jayne got me out of the house. We didn't do much, but by this point, a short trip to a nearby Safeway and People's Drugs was a major adventure. I felt fine after my excursion, and that made us both feel good.

I was up early on Thursday, walking again. My pulse went from 84 to 114 and back to 90 after my exercise. Two weeks after my attack, I spent my first time alone. Jayne and the boys went to the pool in the development. It was only about two minutes away, and they called twice in two hours to make sure I was all right, but it was important for all of us to see that I was fine on my own.

This was the day I went for the short treadmill stress test that I hadn't been able to do at the hospital. It went well. I was supposed to get my heart rate up to 120. It went to 118 with no shortness of breath and no problems with blood pressure. This was more good news, and with each small victory, Jayne and I both felt better.

The next few days were fairly uneventful. On Friday, my last respite friend was Dick Daw, the director at National Catholic News Service. Dick told me about his own scare a few years ago when he ended up in the hospital with chest pains. It seems everyone has a story.

I alternated between good and bad times, often on the same day. In addition to apprehension, I felt guilt and pressure, and I wasn't even sure why. I guess everyone who comes down with a disease that's in any way preventable must feel that same guilt. But, again, it wasn't all bad, even then; my total diary entry for June 30 reads, "Pool, pasta, better."

I was trying to find a balance. On the one hand, I wanted to do a little more every day than I had the day before; I felt that that meant I was making progress. On the other hand, I was very aware that I could do some damage by pressing too much, and I knew it was important to stop when I felt tired. Of course, in walking that tightrope, I put more pressure on myself.

On July 1, I was pooped and slept more than I had in weeks. All that sleep must have done me some good, because I felt terrific the next day. When I went walking, my pulse rate only went up to 96 with the same exertion that had raised it higher just a few days before. After five minutes, it was down to 78, six beats lower than when I had started. I'd never been an exercise freak, to put it mildly, but I knew enough to know that my heart, which is, after all, a muscle, was getting stronger.

I felt good enough to start thinking about work again. I

went down to the office to start straightening out my desk
and go through my mail. I went crazy for a while because
I couldn't find an important file. After searching all over,
I found it in my briefcase. I'd left it there the day before
my attack, a time that now seemed light-years in the past.

After a heart attack, you don't worry only about survival; you worry about work. Will you be able to do your
job? What changes will you have to make? At one level, I
wasn't worried because my job didn't involve heavy physical pressures—I didn't work construction, and I didn't
spend 100 days a year on the road. Essentially, as long as
I could read, use a telephone, and type, I'd be OK.

But there is more to what I do than that. I have to deal
with constant deadline pressure, constant competitive
pressure, and constant pressure to produce and create. I
didn't yet know how I could handle these pressures or
what I'd do if I couldn't.

I had already started a work transition that would help
in some ways but perhaps not in others. Until the past six
months, I had lived with deadlines. After I graduated
from Iona College in New Rochelle, New York, in 1969, I
began work as a journalist, first in New York, then in
Kansas City, Missouri. In 1974, we had come to Washington. I wrote primarily about religious and political issues, and I had spent a lot of time in the Catholic press; I
joked that I seemed destined to explain the church to the
world and the world to the church—and there was plenty
of work.

I was religion editor at *The Washington Star*, one of the
district's two daily papers, when it folded in August 1981.
The closing took me by surprise, and I decided then that
I didn't want to put all my eggs in one basket anymore. I
put together a package of free-lance writing jobs.

I had done just about every kind of writing there was—
news, features, editorials, columns. Over the years, I'd
worked on some stories I was really proud of. In the early
'70s, I'd followed up on a tip from a subscriber at *National*

Catholic Reporter and ended up with a story about how Pope Pius XI had commissioned an encyclical letter condemning racism and anti-semitism in the late 1930s but had died before he could release it; Pius XII had killed the letter. That story made headlines all over the country. I'd written a lot of good stories for *The Washington Star*; one editor said I was the first religion editor they had who could write on deadline; another said I had the instincts of a police reporter.

While I still did some news writing, I was now working with People for the American Way (PFAW), a public interest group, writing reports and newspaper columns, and planning strategy. I had written one book, *The Bishops and the Bomb*, the story of the making of the U.S. bishops' 1983 pastoral letter on peace, and was now working on several books simultaneously. I was writing a profile of American Catholics with George Gallup, Jr., an authorized history of the Campaign for Human Development (the U.S. Catholic bishops' anti-poverty program), and a book on religion and politics for PFAW. It felt good to have fewer deadlines, but I was still feeling my way around a new way of writing.

Whatever kind of writing I did, though, I knew I needed to learn how to relax. In the grand scheme of things, that meant a whole series of attitude adjustments. Most prescriptions for relaxation techniques begin with something like this: "Go to a dark, quiet room for a half hour." If you have a dark, quiet room to yourself for a half hour, you could relax well enough without meditation. I never seemed to have that luxury. I needed something that would bring me down quickly, like a tranquilizer dart, in the middle of the day.

But the material I had been given in the hospital included descriptions of two relaxation procedures to use for quick results. One will sound familiar to everyone. Just lie down, tighten all the muscles in your body, and then slowly relax them. Begin with your scalp, then your eyes, then your jaw, and work your way down to your feet, relaxing the muscles one at a time. The second method is the "Relaxation Response" described by Dr. Herbert Benson. It involves simply sitting quietly and concentrating on one point while repeating a soothing sound—that's where the clichéd "MMMMMMMMMM" sound of a mantra comes from. If your mind wanders, focus it back. (Dr. Dean Ornish gives this advice: "Wait a few hours after eating. Meditation increases the blood flow to your brain. Eating increases the blood flow to your digestive system. Choose one or the other."

Learning how to relax was particularly important to me because I had decided that I was a coronary-prone Type A personality. The description came from two doctors, Meyer Friedman and Ray H. Rosenman, who had found a link between a particular personality type and heart disease. In their book, *Type A Behavior and Your Heart*, they said Type A could be found in anyone "who is *aggressively* involved in a *chronic, incessant* struggle to achieve more and more in less and less time, and if required to do so, against the opposing efforts of other things or other persons. . . . Persons possessing this pattern also are quite prone to exhibit a free-floating but extraordinarily well-rationalized hostility."* They said a person is a Type A if he or she struggles to do things faster and faster, chronically tries to think about or do two or more things at a time, anguishes while waiting on line, or feels guilty when relaxing. Friedman and Rosenman defined the benign Type B personality as pretty much the exact opposite of Type A. I thought some of the descriptions were a little extreme, although the authors did concede that there are degrees of Type A personality. However, I saw enough that was familiar in the description of Type A that I didn't question the basic

*From Meyer Friedman, M.D. and Ray H. Rosenman, M.D., *Type A Behavior and Your Heart* (New York: Alfred A. Knopf, 1974) p. 67.

premise. I could see that, when push came to shove, I easily qualified as a Type A.

As I settled in at home and the shock of the attack continued to wear off, a new wave of apprehension set in. I had agreed to have an angiogram in another few weeks, but as Jayne and I talked about it, we saw that we were both nervous about the procedure. This was the first time I realized it was completely elective, and I began wondering whether I should elect it. Jayne's father had died during an angiogram following a heart attack. Though our situations were not similar—he was 76—Jayne's anxiety was understandable. Even though the risk was fairly low, neither one of us was eager to take on any more risk at all. I thought the procedure wasn't necessary unless I developed other symptoms. I decided to get some outside advice and called Dr. Edmund Pellegrino, now the head of the Kennedy Center for Ethics at Georgetown University. I had met him when he was president of Catholic University; he was a physician specializing in cardiac issues.

The next day, I did some actual work for the first time. For my book on the history of the bishops' anti-poverty program, I had been trying to reach Cardinal Joseph Bernardin of Chicago. He had been a key figure in the program's creation in the late '60s. A secretary from his office called on the morning of July 3 and asked if I'd be able to do a telephone interview. We did the interview, and I got the information I needed. He asked how I felt, and I said I felt fine. I still don't know whether he knew about my attack, and I didn't see any need to bring it up. Whether he knew or not, just doing that little bit of work was good for my morale.

But the roller-coaster ride continued. The Fourth of July started out fine; we cooked out in the back yard. But Jayne and I were up until 1:30 in the morning talking. We were still in our vicious circle. I was still closed off, but my feelings were starting to break through. Of course, the first feelings to come out were unfocused anger and guilt. It wasn't pleasant, but it was a start.

Dr. Pellegrino called back the next day, and he was very reassuring about the angiogram. He helped me ask the right questions about the procedure's risks and the benefits; the risks were small, and the benefits were great. The angiogram, he said, was the only way to learn the "geography of the lesion" and see if my heart could withstand another attack. My doctors had called the angiogram "the gold standard," and I finally accepted it. On July 9, I made an appointment to have an angiogram on July 18.

In my conversation with Dr. Pellegrino, I told him about the "heart attack flu" episode I'd had two and a half years ago. One of my doctors had recently looked back at the records of that incident and had said my EKG suggested some problem, and I told Dr. Pellegrino about it. I came away from our conversation convinced that there had been a problem back then that had been missed— and convinced that if it had been picked up two-and-a-half years ago, I wouldn't have had my heart attack.

This information was a bombshell; Jayne and I talked, and I contacted a malpractice lawyer. But I talked to Dr. Pellegrino again a few days later to make sure I had understood him correctly; I hadn't. He didn't see any grounds for a suit. More important, he said, the pressure and stress of such a suit would hurt my recovery, which was far more important. I saw that he was right; I was having trouble coping with mere day-to-day stress right now, and the demands of a lawsuit would be just too much. This would be particularly true if I didn't have a rock-solid case. I dropped the idea. As it turned out, there is a two-year statute of limitations for medical malpractice suits in Virginia, and I wouldn't have been able to sue even if I had a clear-cut case. I suspect that my reaction was typical. A lawsuit would have given me someone other than myself to blame for my attack.

My guilt feelings were particularly high at that point. At the time of my heart attack, I was still covered under a benefits package from my old job. Benefits included a good-sized life insurance policy, but my coverage had run out on June 30. I had let getting more insurance slide; it's not something most people want to think about, and I guess I figured that at 38 I didn't have to worry about dying very soon. As a result, I now found myself with a wife, two children, a badly damaged heart, an uncertain future, and only a small life insurance policy from a few years back. Of course, I had no prospect of getting more insurance in a hurry. I was trying to get out of my emotional box, but I felt as if I were repeatedly getting pushed back into it.

The anxiety produced by the life insurance situation was intensified by current financial problems. Not surprisingly, given the situation, more money than usual was going out, less was coming in, and other money that eventually would come in would be delayed because I'd be late in finishing the work. Focusing on this was draining, but Jayne realized that there was a reason we spent so much time talking about finances: the subject, at least, was tangible—we could get our hands on it. Jayne was also going through something common to others in her situation. She'd been working part-time as a secretary at nearby George Mason University and was thinking about taking a full-time job. Because of my heart attack, she was convinced it was necessary to help financially in case I couldn't do what I'd done before.

On the Saturday after the Fourth, I made my first excursion to a shopping mall since my attack. The trip was tiring, but I bounced back faster than I expected. I was feeling pretty good. That must have boosted my confidence. Up to then, Jayne and I had done some very tentative snuggling but had respected the doctors' directive to not resume "relations" until my one-month checkup, which was still about a week away. The doctors had done a good job of persuading me that sex after a heart attack was OK; unlike many men who've had heart attacks, I wasn't afraid of post-attack sex. But lust wasn't the motivator; what Jayne and I needed was intimacy. So we didn't wait for the one-month checkup, and I'm glad we didn't.

July is a month of family celebrations for us. The tenth was Matt's fifteenth birthday, and we took the boys to Matt's favorite seafood restaurant so he could have his favorite, crab legs. The thirteenth was our seventeenth wedding anniversary, and Jayne and I went out for dinner and a drink. There was, however, a feeling of apprehension at both celebrations.

On a lighter note, we were having fun experimenting with cooking "heart-smart" foods. I had never been much of a cook, but I started cooking a lot myself, and it was fun and relaxing. We had *The American Heart Association Cookbook* and *The Don't Eat Your Heart Out Cookbook*. We also had *Heart Smart*, a cookbook published by the people who make Promise margarine. There were some disasters. Tofu banana cream pie didn't get rave reviews, and I don't think I'll ever be sick enough to eat brown rice again. A recipe for a Middle Eastern bean pie, made with chickpeas and sesame seeds, turned out to be what we knew in New York as knishes. They were delicious, but the bean paste left total mayhem in the kitchen. However, Jayne still asks for my high-grain pizza, and I love the pasta stew from *Heart Smart*.

One evening, I called my Aunt Lena in New York. At the time, she was in her late '70s and had severe angina. (She later had a successful triple bypass at age 81.) We talked about diet and changes. She said a friend saw her drinking skim milk and said, "But I don't like skim milk." Lena said, "I don't like it either, but I drink it because I have to."

After being home almost a month and eating nothing but healthful food, I decided I was entitled to a real steak, especially if I had a lean one. Jayne and I went to a local steak place, Squire Rockwell's, and enjoyed steak, baked potato (no butter or sour cream), and salad. While we were eating, a man and two women sat at a table near us. Each one was at least 75 pounds overweight. They ordered prime rib and baked potatoes piled high with butter and sour cream. They had cheesecake for dessert. It was all I could do not to jump up and say, "Don't you know what you're doing to yourselves?" I knew what they were doing; I'd eaten a meal or two like that in my time.

My work was starting to return to normal, and I talked to some people I hadn't spoken to in a while. I talked to Bill Bole, the Washington correspondent for Religious News Service. He said he'd called the hospital to get a report on my condition, and had gotten the impression that a lot of people had been calling; the operator had said, "Oh, him, he's fine." As I told Bill what had happened, about Willie, and my calling Jayne from my office phone—he said, "Yeah, I heard the story." I was glad people were concerned but I figured I'd earned the right to tell my story myself. I told Bill "You may have heard it but you're going to hear it again."

I called Monsignor Dan Hoye, then general secretary of the National Conference of Catholic Bishops, to thank him for asking the bishops to pray for me at their meeting. Hoye was only a year or two older than I, and I had had a soft spot for him since I interviewed him when he was appointed. I asked him what he did for relaxation. Unlike most "leaders" I'd interviewed, who tend to say they listen to classical music and read biographies of Winston Churchill, Hoye admitted that he relaxed by sailing and reading Robert Ludlum-style thrillers. When I thanked him, he joked, "When they told me about your attack, they also said you were 'lucid,' but I wasn't going to try to convince anyone of that." When I told him the Southern Baptists had also been praying for me, he said,

"Well, they prayed more literally, and we prayed more transcendently."

I got a nice note from Archbishop John Foley, the Vatican's communications director. I had known John when he was the editor of the Catholic newspaper in Philadelphia, and he was a good guy. He suggested that I write about my experience, saying I could help bring people closer to God. I wrote to thank him for his note, and said I wasn't going to write about my experience just yet. I told him I'd been as close to God as I wanted to get for a while.

I thought a lot about religion during this period. How could I not? I laughed a little at the irony: I had religious leaders praying for me, but I hadn't asked for a chaplain in the hospital. Even though I had spent most of my career covering religion or dealing with religion in some fashion, I hadn't been to church, except for work or weddings, since an anti-war Mass on campus in 1966. I sometimes joke that I belong to the second-largest religious denomination in the country—lapsed Catholics. There are more of us than there are Southern Baptists.

I've never been much of a joiner, and I don't have a liturgical bone in my body. I guess, if pressed, I'd call myself a believing agnostic. I'm very pragmatic. Can we prove the existence or nonexistence of God? No. We believe what we want to believe. I choose to believe there's a God, something bigger than we are, something that will eventually produce justice. I believe there are no atheists in foxholes, and I felt as if I were in a foxhole now.

When you ask, "Why did this happen to me?" or "Why did I survive?" you're asking a theological question. I didn't have any answers. When I came home from the hospital, I asked Jayne to buy me a copy of Thornton Wilder's *The Bridge of San Luis Rey*, about a monk who tried to find out why a group of travelers who died together in an accident died when they did. But I never did reread it.

I was surprised how often my doctors, people of science, talked about God. When I mentioned that I hadn't had any problems with allergies since my attack, even though it was my peak allergy season, Dr. Marder said, "God's giving you a break." When I told Dr. Bhushan about my concern regarding the angiogram, he said, "Things are going your way so far; this will go your way. There were plenty of chances for you to die. God wants you to live a long, long time."

I was a little more comfortable with Dr. Herron's approach. He said, "You have to play the cards the way they're dealt." I didn't see that I had much choice. Agonizing over why the cards were dealt the way they were wasn't going to help me play my hand. People who have a deep faith usually find comfort in it during a time of illness. But the way I worked was to focus on the job at hand and do it.

I saw Dr. Bhushan for a checkup on July 11, and he said that in four and a half years at Fairfax Hospital, he hadn't lost any of his patients during an angiogram. He said the death rate for the procedure at the hospital was one in a thousand, which was impressive. I'd read that the death rate nationally was about one in three hundred to four hundred.

I told Dr. Bhushan I was still experiencing chest pain, and he put me on a new medication, Isordil. This, like the Procardia, was supposed to dilate blood vessels to keep my blood flowing smoothly. I didn't feel any chest pain when I walked the next day, so I thought it might be helping.

At this point, I called Jim Metcalf to get more detailed information about NOVACAT. He described it as a 16-week, 32-session program, after which the patient could continue on a "maintenance" basis. At each session, Mondays and Thursdays, patients weigh in and get their blood pressure checked, do some stretching and other exercises, and walk or jog for 20–30 minutes. Each session usually ended with a film or lecture. He said patients needed to fulfill three criteria to begin the program: they had to have cardiovascular disease, they had to have passed the eight-week treadmill test, and they had to have a doctor's recommendation. I would have no problem meeting these requirements.

In looking forward to NOVACAT, I found myself thinking about a friend who had died the previous fall, Geno Baroni, a Catholic priest and "activist." Geno was a colorful figure who told a lot of great stories; some of them actually happened. He had grown up in the coal country in Pennsylvania. After he was ordained, he became a "labor priest" and spent a great deal of his time supporting the labor movement and protecting workers' rights. By the '60s, Geno had relocated to Washington, D.C., and had become a leader in the civil rights movement. He was a friend of Bobby Kennedy and was active in his presidential campaign.

By the late '60s, Geno realized that many of the problems facing urban blacks were the same problems that faced their white neighbors, who were mostly working-class Catholic ethnics—Poles, Italians, Slavs, and so on. Geno was one of the first to lead an "urban ethnic" movement; while others exploited black-ethnic tensions, Geno worked to undo them. He worked on neighborhood development issues, and eventually he became the first priest to serve in a sub-cabinet position in the federal government. Jimmy Carter had named Geno an assistant secretary of Housing and Urban Development. (Geno's friends recall the story about his first meeting with Carter during the 1976 presidential campaign. Geno came away saying that Carter was a little "strange"; we speculated about what the born-again southern peanut farmer might have thought about Geno.)

Geno was by nature an organizer, and he faced his greatest challenge in the early '80s. It was then that he learned that something he had been exposed to in the mines had given him a rare form of cancer, and that it was terminal. Geno, the apostle of neighborhood self-help groups, looked around and discovered self-help groups in the health area as well. He worked with and got help from some cancer self-help groups. He became an apostle of these groups as well, until the day he died. In thinking about Geno, I realized even more forcefully that I was going to have to help myself—and that I'd have to get help from others who had been through the same thing I had.

As a writer, I knew the difference between being "eager" to do something and being "anxious" to do it. "Eager" means you are looking forward to it; "anxious" means you have anxiety about it. I was both eager and anxious to start NOVACAT. When Matt was a baby, we read that babies go through stages when they cry a lot for no apparent reason. This happens because their minds have developed faster than their bodies; their minds can envision doing things that their bodies can't do yet. That's just how I felt.

And I was definitely "anxious" about the angiogram. I had come almost full circle. Now I wanted it done as soon as possible so I could find out exactly what I was dealing with. By the day before the procedure, Jayne and I were both in terrible shape. She was convinced I was going to die *during* the procedure, and I was convinced I was going to die *before* it.

4

STRUGGLE

We began the day of my angiogram bright and early. I had to be at the hospital for prepping—and general waiting—several hours before the procedure. I talked to my roommate, who was about to go home after a balloon angioplasty. He said that as soon as the balloon was inflated and had flattened out his blockage, he felt a rush of oxygen to his brain and a burst of energy.

The first prepping step was a shave. My roommate Denny at Commonwealth had told me a funny story about his shaving experience. He said a big black orderly built something like Rosey Grier came in brandishing a straight razor and said, "I's going to shave your groins now." Denny thought he was a goner. But the guy actually gave him a good, gentle shave. I should have been suspicious, then, when a short, white orderly with bookish-looking glasses came in and asked about the Barbara Tuchman book Jayne had brought to read while she was waiting. He pulled out what felt like a used disposable razor and proceeded to nick the hell out of me. This was not an auspicious beginning.

I was supposed to rest and get an IV for two hours before the procedure, but the operating room was backed up and we got started late. Waiting is the thing I do worse than anything else in the world, and the more important the event I'm waiting for, the worse I am. Jayne and I have two completely different ways of dealing with impending crises. She's a nervous wreck in anticipation, but calm during the crisis itself. I'm fairly calm beforehand, but my anxiety peaks during the crisis. One of us is always a wreck, but, on the bright side, one of us is always in control.

I was finally brought down to the operating room. The whole procedure would be recorded on videotape. I was given one last opportunity to empty my bladder before the doctors started—I was assured that it wouldn't be on the tape. Dr. Marder, who was going to do the angiogram, asked if I wanted any particular music; they had assembled quite a tape library. I said I often listened to Willie Nelson's *Stardust* album when I needed to relax, and I could use that now. Later on, when I told Jayne that story, she choked up. She said that when the doctors hadn't expected me to live, she had planned to play that album at my funeral. They didn't have *Stardust* in the operating room, but they did play my country station on the radio.

They placed one catheter in my arm and another one in my groin. My groin had been shot full of Novocain™ first, but it still hurt. They have to put a lot of pressure on the groin to prevent blood from spurting out. If they didn't, Marder said, I could "exsanguinate"—what a lovely word!

As the procedure began, I began to faint. My blood pressure fell quickly to something like 70 over 40. They gave me some medication through the catheter in my arm, and I felt fine. Marder, who knew that Jayne had been upset about the angiogram, said, "Your wife made a nervous wreck of you." I told him not to blame her because I was capable of getting pretty nervous all by myself. He said, "Let's just say a wreck was made."

I felt pretty much what I had been told I would feel during the actual procedure—some hot flashes and some chest pain. A TV monitor showed exactly what the injected dye was finding, but I didn't have my glasses on, so I couldn't really see it. I don't know whether I would have understood it.

When the procedure was done, I was wheeled into a recovery room where a nurse put a clamp on the groin incision. An orderly stood over me, pressing down on the incision for a full hour. That's standard procedure to make sure it heals properly—and that you don't exsanguinate.

By the time I got back to my room, Jayne was considerably less calm from the long wait. We had to wait even longer for Marder to get back with the results.

The results read like a good news–bad news joke. First, we heard the good news. Marder said that although doctors generally talk about the three main arteries to the heart, about 40 percent of the population actually has a different configuration. In this configuration, the right artery is practically vestigial, like an appendix, and the left artery is double size and does double duty. That was the configuration I had. We knew the front artery was blocked. My right artery was completely blocked, but it was so small that it hadn't been doing me any good before it was blocked. And the left artery—Jayne and I immediately dubbed it "Superartery"—was "clean as a whistle." There were no blockages in it and no need for a bypass or angioplasty. I asked what the risk of another heart attack was, and Marder said, "Practically none," an unusually upbeat assessment from any doctor.

Then came the bad news. The angiogram had also revealed a ventricular aneurism. This is essentially a flap of tissue that remained alive in the damaged area of my heart. The aneurism would use blood and oxygen to stay alive, without doing me any good. Marder said the aneurism could cause serious problems, but it was hard to tell because they were looking at "a two-dimensional picture of a three-dimensional object." What did all that mean? "You won't see 65," he said. But he said he'd had patients with an aneurism who were doing fine after five years. I had liked Marder when I was at Commonwealth Hospital because he was upbeat; now I found he was just as flip with bad news as he was with good.

I tried to tell Marder that what he said didn't make sense. I had walked a half-mile at a fairly brisk pace the day before without any symptoms, and my heart had responded just fine. Surely if the aneurism were going to create a problem, the problem would have shown up by now. But we were having two different conversations, and he didn't even seem to hear me.

When he left, Jayne and I were devastated. We both felt we'd been told that I was going to be a cripple for four or five years and then die. I needed some rest, Jayne needed to get home to the boys, and we both needed to reassess our situation.

I called the cardiac unit at Commonwealth Hospital to get input from some of the nurses I knew there. They said that what Marder said sounded extreme, and that if I weren't satisfied, I should call him. My nurse at Fairfax said the same thing. I called and left a message. When Marder called back that evening and I pressed him, it was like talking to a different person than I'd talked to that afternoon.

Marder said that when he said I wouldn't see 65, he was reflecting statistics that show that a person who has had a heart attack generally has a shorter life span than other people. He said that the statistics said nothing about me personally and that the object of the care I'd be receiving was "to bring the curve up."

I asked him why he had talked about patients doing fine with an aneurism for only five years. He said that that was how long he'd been treating them. They were still doing fine. I asked if the fact that they were doing fine after five years meant they'd probably continue to do fine. Marder said it did.

Then I asked what, specifically, I should look for if the aneurism did cause a problem. The first symptom, he said, was chest pain, a minor problem. The second symptom was shortness of breath. He said my activities would be restricted. If I did heavy lifting for a living, I'd have to change jobs. "If you play softball with your kids, you won't be able to run to first base." Marder said if this became a real problem, there was the possibility of surgery to remove or sew over the aneurism.

The third possible problem was arrhythmia, irregular heart rhythms. They could monitor for this, Marder said, and, if they found it, there were plenty of medications for it.

Marder said I was on "hardly any medication at all," and the fact that I didn't even need a diuretic showed that my heart could handle pumping the fluids it needs to pump. He said an exercise program would help compensate for the flap.

I called Jayne immediately after this conversation, and we both felt an incredible sense of relief. Now what we were working with made sense and wasn't nearly as threatening.

When I woke up the next day, I felt as if I had a third lease on life. Marder said that, because I was doing OK so far, I'd probably continue to do fine. He said I should have a stress test and a heart monitor once a year and shouldn't lose touch with my doctors.

Later that day, I thought about my flap. It was a piece of tissue that should have died but didn't. I could relate. After all, I thought, what was I?

Even though I felt considerably better than I had the

night before, I knew I still had plenty of unfinished business. But when I went home, two domestic crises gave me good reminders that the world hadn't stood still just because I'd had a heart attack. First, our car broke down again and had to go back to the dealer for servicing. Then Willie suddenly started walking with a severe limp on his front left leg. It scared us all; Jayne and I knew the boys would be heartbroken if something happened to Willie.

Our vet kept him overnight for observation and did some X-rays. The news was good—he just had the canine version of growing pains and would be OK. I took him for a walk when we got him home. Jayne watched us, me limping on my right leg from the incision and Willie limping on his left, and said, "The two of you look like Charlie Chaplin walking down the street."

Dan was upset that day. Even though we had explained that I was just going back in the hospital for a test, he was still afraid and told me, "I thought you were going to die." He felt better after I talked to him some more. Dan and I usually eat breakfast together, and he became my conscience when it came to skim milk; if on occasion we ran out and I poured some two percent milk on my Cheerios, he gave me a hard time.

By later that day, I actually started to feel normal for the first time. The next day I had a good walk—a half-mile, with my pulse going from 93 to 111 and back to 93 in five minutes. But I was bored and restless. Something was brewing, and I was an absolute maniac the day after that. I burned some muffins I was making in the morning and took my frustration out on everyone else all day long.

I worked half a day in the morning. I increased my walk to three-quarters of a mile, which I did in 12 minutes. I talked to Jim Metcalf about my aneurism. He said he didn't have any experience with them, but that the premise that exercise would help made sense.

But I was restless and feeling cooped up after dinner. I blew up and screamed at the boys, kicked open the door to Dan's room, and ran out of the house. I just walked and sat in the nearby bus stop shed, occasionally talking to neighbors, for about 40 minutes. When I came back, everyone was upset. Jayne had looked for me and couldn't find me, so she was naturally worried about me—while, of course, still being rightfully angry. I made up with Dan that night, but I was still having trouble talking to Matt and asked Jayne for help. Sometimes Matt and I are so alike that we can't communicate at all. I told Jayne that night that I was going stir-crazy—I needed to know what I could do, and I still didn't know.

I was able to talk to Matt the next day. Like Dan, he was going through a delayed fear reaction to my attack, but he felt better after we talked. It's funny, but I can't remember just what I said. It seems that simply talking about your fears may be as important as what you actually say.

I worked a half-day again and had a good walk, but the news on the automotive front wasn't good. I was doing fine, but our mechanic said the car had only eight or ten weeks to live. It was definitely trade-in time, and we spent the next couple of days looking at new cars.

We ended up back at the Ford place, figuring they owed us a good deal after what we had gone through with the Escort. I didn't think that they had anything in the size we wanted, but the Thunderbird was now a family-size car. They had two 1985 models for sale equipped the way we wanted, a white one and a red one. We asked to look at the white one because it was a little cheaper, but the salesman brought the red one over. It wasn't just red—it was fire engine red. It was an anniversary model marking the thirtieth year of the Thunderbird, and it came loaded with everything you could think of. Sitting in the front seats was like sitting in the waiting room of a fancy lawyer. We took it for a test drive, fell in love with it, and bought it. Jayne looked great driving it, and I thought we deserved a little luxury. I said, "Hey, this is the kind of car you buy when you have a heart attack and live."

The whole process took several hours and we had started after dinner, so I was exhausted, but I felt fine in the morning. I was beginning to develop some endurance again. While we were at the dealer, we heard the heart story of one of the salesmen. He had been driving to work when he went completely numb on one side of his body. He managed to drive himself to a hospital, get out of the car, and crawl into the emergency room with his one usable arm and leg. The doctors did a triple bypass, and he was back at work. Of course, when we saw him, he was eating a couple of bacon cheeseburgers. Some people never learn; some people who survive a heart attack seem to think they're immortal and go about tempting the gods.

Jayne and I had a good talk the day before we bought the car. I thanked her for putting up with my intensity about recovery. She had made several references to my having "a bad heart," and I asked her to stop. I had a "damaged heart" or a "heart condition," I said, but to me the term "bad heart" meant one on the brink that couldn't take very much work or strain. That wasn't the case with me. She said she understood, and then she helped me deal better with something else that had bothered me. I had found when talking to people after my attack that they often asked a lot of stupid questions, and I started to get annoyed. Jayne said people asked stupid questions because the situation was scary, and they just needed to say something. I became much more tolerant.

About this time, someone asked us what we'd learned from our experience, and it was useful to be reflective. Jayne said she'd learned that she needed to be more independent, more able to take care of herself. This was one reason she had decided to work full time instead of part time. She had applied for a new job as receptionist and secretary in the psychological counseling office at George Mason University, and we were now waiting to hear whether she would get it.

I began to realize how much Jayne loved me; I had never doubted it, but I really felt it in a new way now. I also learned two important things. First, it is possible—not easy, but possible—to change from a Type A personality to a Type B and slow down. Second, emotional stress is much worse than physical exertion; it really takes a toll. If you're physically tired, you can feel better after a good night's sleep. But stress can go on forever, feeding on itself and multiplying.

By the end of July, I realized that I was going hours at a time without thinking about my heart. Taking pills, walking, and eating were regular reminders, but I wasn't dwelling on the situation.

My next medical examination was for the purpose of having my heart rhythms checked by wearing a Holter monitor. (I thought the doctor was saying "halter," and that it was so named because the patient wore it; actually, the device was named for its inventor, Holter.) The monitor was about the size of a very early portable radio. It was hooked up to my chest like an EKG machine, and strapped around my waist with a canvas belt. The monitor contained a miniature tape recorder, which would record every heartbeat during a 24-hour period. The tape would reveal whether there were any irregularities. I hated the Holter. I felt trapped by it, carrying it around all day. It made me feel as if I were back in the hospital. It was hard to sleep with the monitor on my night table because it restricted my movement. But I got through the day and night, dropped it off at the doctor's office, and waited for the results.

The last week of July was an entertaining one. Early in the spring, we had bought tickets for some concerts that all fell in the same week, and we decided to use them. We went twice to Wolf Trap in Vienna, Virginia, for country music—Janie Fricke and the Statler Brothers—and once to the Kennedy Center for Tom Jones.

At Wolf Trap, the seats were almost a mile from the parking lot, and it was all straight uphill. The first time, I took a couple of nitroglycerin pills and felt OK, but the second time, I used the little bus they had for the elderly and handicapped. (Jayne had gotten a handicapped parking sticker that was good for 60 days. I felt funny about using it now that I was walking much longer distances for exercise, but it saved a lot of walking in the Washington heat and humidity. Besides, Jayne said it made up for all the times that she had to walk the whole length of a mall parking lot while pregnant.)

The Janie Fricke concert was great, and when it was over, she and her opening act, Exile, set up shop to sign autographs and sell souvenirs. We went through the line, and I told Janie Fricke I had a complaint—she hadn't sung my favorite among her hits, "Don't Worry 'Bout Me Baby." She said the song's title line for me, and I kissed her hand in thanks. Jayne came up behind carrying an Exile "Woke Up in Love" T-shirt and said, "Is he giving you a hard time because you didn't sing his song?" It was some badly needed fun.

I continued to walk every day, and by the beginning of August, I was walking more than a mile a day. Typically, my pulse would start at about 75, go up to 105, and drop down quickly to 75. There was already a great improvement in my resting pulse rate, the rate first thing in the morning. The lower this rate, the better. Mine was almost 100 when I came home from the hospital, so my heart was now about 25 percent stronger.

I hadn't had any formal exercise training at this point, so I was pretty much winging it. I walked a certain distance until my exercise pulse rate seemed to level off, and then I walked another quarter- or half-mile. We live on a circle that measures a quarter-mile around, so it was easy to measure how much I was walking by counting the number of laps. I put on a Walkman radio or tape player as I walked. I enjoyed the music, and I found I walked in time to it. One day the country music I'd been using felt too slow, and I put on some Springsteen to rev it up. My next-door neighbor, Todd Jacobs, was in training for the Iron Man Decathlon in Hawaii, and he gave me a lot of encouragement. I told him how my pulse was behaving, and he said it sounded as if my heart were responding as well as it should.

Walking proved to be good for my psyche as well as my body. There were many mornings that I started out in a bad mood or angry about something, and felt much better after I had walked for a while. To make it easier to take my pulse while I walked, I ordered a "pulse watch" from a mail order company. I was supposed to put my index finger on a button and it was supposed to tell me my heart rate, but I'd get readings like "32, 225, 70, 49, 197." The instructions said readings might sometimes be off because of electrical interference. Matt said, "Yeah, somebody else's heart must be beating."

The first two days of August brought some good news. On the first, Jayne learned that she had gotten her new job and would start in a couple of weeks. On the second, I got the results of the Holter monitor—everything was fine. I had five extra beats all day, perfectly within the normal range. That eliminated one possible major problem.

But good news never seemed to last long. On August 3, Dan fell off his bike and injured his hand. We took him to the emergency room to get patched up. It was the same emergency room where I'd been treated for my attack. It was a little spooky, but I felt upbeat. While we were there, I saw Dr. Bhushan, so I went over to say hello. I thought he'd be upbeat, too, because I knew that Dr. Herron's office had sent him the Holter report. But instead, I got doom and gloom.

He said, "We'll do the best we can under the circumstances." Then he told me that, because of my age, I was an excellent candidate for a heart transplant if I needed one. He said that because of the aneurism, I'd have to take it easy. I thought that if I took it easy, I'd soon be dead, because I needed to get my heart as strong as possible. And even though my heart was damaged, I was just getting to know it—the idea of having it yanked out didn't appeal to me. I tend to be a fainter, and that brief discussion cut the legs out from under me. I lay down on a bed to regain my equilibrium, and Jayne looked up just in time to see me stretched out.

I was fine in a minute, but the episode was really upsetting. It seemed that every time I took a few steps forward, someone tried to push me back again. The next morning, I walked two miles for the first time; my pulse went from 75 to 114 and back to 84. Even though that was a good workout, I still wasn't happy. I'd taken a different route to cover the extra distance, but I'd consciously avoided the hills—I didn't want to put too much strain on my heart. But that didn't feel right.

I had that feeling again when I went out to walk the next morning. It reminded me of a feeling I'd had almost 20 years before. I've never lived the kind of life that required much in the way of physical bravery—I hadn't been in the military, I wasn't a police officer or a firefighter. I'd mouthed off to a drunk or two in my younger days, but that wasn't bravery; that was just stupidity.

I thought about one day in the summer of 1967. I was in college, and I worked summers, weekends, and holidays at King's, a men's clothing store in Mt. Vernon, New York, where I'd grown up. (I remember that summer well for another reason: Jayne and I started to date. Jayne and I had met in high school several years before, although we take pains to point out that we were not "high school sweethearts"; in fact, we didn't even get along particularly well in high school. We met again a few years later. Here's how it happened: at King's, the employees' favorite pastime on slow Saturday mornings was to stand in front of the store and watch the girls go by. One morning Jayne was one of those girls; we talked, had lunch, and started dating. We were married after my junior year and her freshman year at State University College of New York at Buffalo.)

But 1967 was also the year of major race riots in several American cities. Mt. Vernon bordered on the Bronx, and for a while, it looked as if the Bronx would blow up, too. If it did, the violence would probably spill over into Mt. Vernon. All of the store owners and employees on Fourth Avenue, the city's main shopping area, were worried about violence and damage, and there were plenty of extra police around, sometimes on rooftops.

There was a lot of talk about "outside agitators" in all of the riot-torn areas. Most of the talk came from people who didn't want to recognize the problems in their own back yards. Still, there was something to it. About half of our customers were black, and they told us they were suddenly seeing a lot of strange faces in town. To complicate matters, the store's manager was doing two weeks of National Guard duty, and I, at age 20, was in charge of the store. I had to open and close the store and take each day's receipts to the bank. There were three of us working, and we weren't a very formidable group: I, with my thick eyeglasses; Al Balzarini, a roly-poly, 64-year-old man who was counting the days until retirement; and Jimmy Reynolds, a tall, skinny, shy young black.

One day when Jimmy was out to lunch, a strange black came into the store, and I could tell he wasn't a regular customer. He just wanted to know where we kept the silk pants and the Italian knit shirts in his size. I figured he wanted to know just where to find his size when he came back that night to loot the store. I hadn't noticed it, but Al said he saw a small open knife in the guy's hand, and Al hovered over me until the guy left.

The tension mounted every day. After about a week of this, I got to the store one morning and saw three or four young black men I didn't know hanging around the lobby in front of the store. In order to open up, I had to walk past them, kneel down, and unlock the front door from the bottom, with my back to them. Everything I'd been hearing the past week—from police, storekeepers, customers—told me not to do it. But I'd just had enough; I thought, "I can't live like this. I've got to do my job."

I walked past them, knelt down, and unlocked the door. They came in, chatted, bought a couple of sport shirts, and left. We never did have a problem. But I remembered that feeling. That was exactly the way I felt now—I couldn't live with myself if I were afraid to walk up a hill. This time, I took a different route that began with a half-mile uphill walk to a nearby lake. The lake was a mile around with several steep hills. I walked at a brisk clip; my pulse went from 75 to 129 and back to 99. This reflected the greater exertion, but it was fine. I felt terrific—and I could look at myself in the mirror again.

I was still upset, however, and I really needed to talk to people to get a different perspective. Our neighbor Ellen said I should talk to people with success stories. To start, I called Mary Simms, a social worker at Fairfax Hospital who worked with cardiac patients. I told her my situation, and I told her about the conflict between the way I felt and the doom and gloom I was getting from Marder and Bhushan.

She had some great insights. First, she said, the rule in cardiac care is that doctors are dealing with the kind of people to whom they can't tell anything. These people are obsessive and resistant to change. The doctors need to come on strong to generate some crucial lifestyle changes. When they get someone like me, she said, who's not resistant, they scare the person to death. Another factor, she said, is that all doctors present the worst-risk scenario. She said she'd gone in to have a small tumor removed from her foot, and by the time she'd heard all the risk factors, she felt as if she'd had both legs amputated above the knees.

She said there was a lot of health in both Jayne and me and that I'd learned a lot about my life and how to develop a more healthful lifestyle. And she agreed that it would be good to talk to other people like us.

As it happened, I'd just heard that someone I knew, Frank Monahan, a lobbyist with the U.S. Catholic Conference, had had a heart attack the previous year. I called Frank to hear his story and get some tips.

Frank is a tall, big, ruddy-faced, gregarious Irishman who was born to be a lobbyist. He told me his attack had come the previous year in Dallas, where he was presenting U.S. Catholic Conference testimony before the Republican National Committee platform hearings. He woke up one morning with a crushing pain in his chest. A colleague drove him to a nearby hospital emergency room. Frank said to me, "I told them this was serious. I wasn't about to take a number and sit down."

The doctors diagnosed a heart attack and stabilized him. He didn't need surgery, but they recommended a lot of rest. Now he was back at work, doing fine. He'd played racquetball before, and he was playing it again. He said his doctors had watched him pretty closely for a year, but they were more relaxed now. "If you make it through the first year," he said, "they don't worry as much."

I learned two important things from Frank. First, he said he'd learned how important it was to get enough rest; if he did that, he felt fine. Second, he said he'd been able to work as well as he had before without being as driven. It was possible to do a good job without being compulsive. The talk was a real pick-me-up. I figured if Frank could learn to slow down, so could I.

Jayne and I had decided it was time to get away for a little bit. We left Matt and Dan with my father and sister for a weekend and drove out to Front Royal, Virginia. But we had a problem when we got there on Friday evening. We took Jayne to the emergency room at the local hospital because she was experiencing excessive menstrual bleeding. The fact was, she had begun her period on the day of my heart attack, and it had never completely stopped. Her doctor had first attributed the problem to the shock of my attack. She had also recently lost a lot of weight, and that could also have thrown off her system. The doctors got things under control in the emergency room, but her problem continued for a year until she had a hysterectomy the following August. But that was all ahead of us at this point.

She felt better the next day. I began with a two-mile walk, and we spent much of the day tromping through Thunderbird Park and Skyline Cavern. The tour of the cavern ends with a climb of almost 100 steps. I took six nitroglycerin pills that day. We went to our first country fair that night and enjoyed it. Jayne's a real animal lover, and she was petting a cow when it stepped on her foot. Luckily, it didn't do any damage. A young boy tried to sell her a raffle ticket to win a pig. "What in the world would I do with a pig?" she asked, and the boy looked at her as if she were an idiot because—his look seemed to say—*everybody* knows what to do with a pig. I was exhausted that evening, but I had a solid eight hours of sleep and bounced back.

When we got back home, I was antsy again. I was due for a checkup with Dr. Herron. My treadmill stress test—the big one—was also coming up. I couldn't shake my anger at Marder and Bhushan, and it was reassuring to see Herron again; he was nice and steady, no peaks and valleys. I saw him for a checkup on August 13, exactly two months after my attack; the stress test was scheduled for two days later.

I seemed to be doing fine. Herron upped the dosage of Isordil because of my chest pain, which he said was probably coming from the "transitional" area around the damaged area in my heart. He said medicine and conditioning would help. Overall, he said, he was an "optimistic realist" about my condition. He likened me to a six-cylinder car running on four cylinders—he said it works if the four cylinders are kept in good shape. He gave me an OK to start at NOVACAT if my stress test showed good results—"You're due to get started," he said.

I asked about the aneurism and possible surgery. He said surgery would be indicated if I had angina or fluid retention that couldn't be controlled by medication, and I didn't have either of those. If surgery ever did become indicated, they would do another catheterization to determine if the problem were operable; if it were inoperable, a transplant was a possibility. But that was all hypothetical right now. He said he thought it was a bad break that someone my age had had that kind of a heart attack. But he said I could look at the glass as either half full or half empty and take it from there—"Play the cards the way they're dealt." I didn't see that I had much choice. I had to see the glass as half full.

Jayne and I felt a little better, but we were still anxious about the stress test. The day finally came. The stress test had three parts. For the first three minutes, I'd walk on a level path at one and a half miles an hour. For the second three minutes, I'd walk a mile an hour faster at an incline. The third three minutes was to be another mile an hour faster at a steeper incline. The goal was to get to my maximum heart rate—220 minus my age, so I had to get to 180 beats per minute—without any problems. I was hooked up to EKG and blood pressure monitors.

Herron described the pace of the first part of the test as like "walking the dog." Thinking of Willie, I asked if that meant stopping every ten feet. As I moved into the second stage, I saw the way he watched the monitors. I was starting to feel the strain, but I was OK. As we moved into the third stage, he kept saying, "This is just to see what you can do. Don't go beyond your limits. You've got nothing to prove." I thought, "Bullshit, I've got nothing to prove," but I didn't say it because I'd given him enough of my complaints two days before.

But as I watched him watch the monitor, I knew the meaning of the expression, "His eyes bugged out of his head." He couldn't believe what he was seeing. "One minute to go," he said, asking me if I needed to stop. No way. At the nine-minute mark, he said, "You got it," and scaled the treadmill down.

I was panting like a racehorse and my chest was killing me, but I felt good. I had gotten my pulse rate to 180 without any sign of heart stress. He gave me a nitroglycerin pill for my chest pain—and it didn't help. That meant the pain I was feeling wasn't heart pain; it wasn't angina. It was either "cardiac neurosis" or muscular-skeletal pain.

"Cardiac neurosis" is a term used to describe a condition in which people either think they have heart trouble when they don't or have it and think it's worse than it really is. I knew I wasn't immune, but it wasn't as if I didn't have people talking about taking out my heart and giving me a new one. This time, at least, I was confident that it wasn't cardiac neurosis. They had beat the hell out of me doing CPR, and that tenderness in bone and cartilage was what I was feeling when I exerted myself.

Herron called it "a terrific stress test." Then he said, "You've got a lot of damage, but the rest of the heart is doing a pretty good job." He said I'd done better than he'd expected. When he brought Jayne in to tell her the results, he got on the treadmill to show her how fast I had been going.

He gave me final approval for NOVACAT and said it would be good for me psychologically—"You've tried so hard." When Jayne and I got into the hall, we jumped and hugged. It was like a graduation. She said it still hurt to hear him talk about how much damage I had. But I'd done better than anyone expected. "I didn't expect bad news," Jayne said. "I thought he'd say, 'That's about what we expected . . .' But not this."

I can't say I expected that good a stress test. I didn't know exactly what to expect. But I knew I was in better shape than anyone else thought I was. I knew I wasn't walking my ass off for nothing. But I thought I deserved an "I told you so." I've never been that high in my life.

5

REHAB

For days after my stress test, I was still flying. But something still wasn't right; there was still an emotional gap between Jayne and me, and we could fight over anything or nothing.

Two days after the stress test, right out of the blue, Jayne yelled at me and I yelled right back. After she went to work, I hurt all day. I felt so distant; I was coming out of my shell, but now it felt as though she were the one doing the withdrawing. Jayne called from work in the afternoon and apologized for the morning. "These feelings surprise me, too," she said. I told her how much I appreciated her call, and I apologized for being short-tempered myself.

That night, we talked again, and I could finally put my feelings into words: "I feel that you're treating me as though I *did* die." She didn't respond right away, but three days later, she said she'd been thinking about what I'd said. "You said I was treating you as though you had died," she said, "and I was. I 'died' you. They told me you were going to die, and I got stuck. And you're so much a part of me that part of me died, too."

That conversation was the breakthrough for me on the emotional level that the stress test had been on a physical level. I was able to see the whole picture again, and I started to feel in a new way the pain that Jayne had been feeling. Jayne never panicked through the whole episode, but she was in a state of emotional shock. We both started to heal—and heal pretty fast—after that night. That night couldn't have happened unless I had had a good stress test. Together, the two events marked the end of convalescence and the beginning of "normal" life.

My new normal life now included a great deal of walking. If walking had gotten me in good enough shape to do that well on the stress test, I was going to keep it up. I was now walking three miles a day in about 39 minutes, getting my pulse rate up to 135. My "target pulse rate"— 80 percent of my maximum pulse rate—was 144, but I rarely got that high. That in itself was a good sign, because it meant that my heart could easily handle my walking at a pretty brisk pace.

The only problem was that my chest and back muscles, which were still sore, had begun to hurt a lot more. I realized that my walking was putting a lot of stress on my legs. This stress was reverberating through my whole body. Jayne said it was time to throw out my old sneakers and graduate to a good pair of running shoes. For someone who had probably never spent more than $13.99 on a pair of sneakers before, it was quite a shock to walk into The Athlete's Foot and see running shoes that cost up to $100. Some were even more. I looked at a couple of styles of walking shoes, but when I told the salesman the way I walked, he said I needed the cushioning of a running shoe. I settled on a pair of Nike Airs that were on sale for a mere $50; I also bought a couple of pairs of thick, cushioned sport socks.

It made a tremendous difference—no more pain. In

fact, just a few days after I got them, I hit my new walking goal. In my laps around the lake, I had been closing in on the 12-minute mile, with times like 12:13 and 12:15. I decided I was going to walk a mile in less than 12 minutes; that's a 5-mph pace. On August 25, about 11 weeks after my heart attack, I did it—a mile in 11:58. Breaking the 4-minute mile never meant more to any runner than breaking the 12-minute mile meant to me. A few months later, with no humidity and the breeze at my back, I did a mile in 10:52.

My work life was approaching normal as well. At the end of August, I started writing my weekly column for Gannett News Service again. I was back in the news flow, and a weekly deadline didn't seem threatening anymore. In late August, *Time* called with an assignment; Jayne said it was good that people weren't leaving me alone, and she was right. August 30 was a big day—my first day going downtown to Washington. There was no reason I couldn't have gone sooner, but there was no reason to go, either, and Washington is no pleasure in the summer under the best of circumstances. The city was built on a swamp, and a swamp it has remained.

I had several appointments, and I promised Jayne I'd check in with her each time I reached one. It got to be a joke, but we both felt better. I had lunch with David Kusnet and Melanne Verveer from People for the American Way, and stopped by the Campaign for Human Development to get some more material for the project I was working on. It was a full day, and it felt good, as if another milestone had been passed.

September was something of a coming-out month. We did more socializing than usual and certainly more than we had the past two months. We went to Willie's "puppy reunion"—a party with his breeder and the owners of some of Willie's brothers and sisters. We went to a Labor Day party with people from Jayne's new office. The party was in the evening of a long day and I was pretty tired; I must have looked awful because everyone told Jayne how tired I looked. She had a hard time convincing them that I really was going well. I decided that if everybody tells you you look tired, you're tired, so I slept late the next day. I must admit, working out of home has some advantages.

In early September, I called an old friend in New York to report in. Bobby Duncan had been my best friend since the first day of junior high school when we both realized simultaneously—and miles ahead of the rest of our class, which was supposed to be the brightest in the grade—that our science teacher was deaf. It opened up interesting possibilities; I'm not proud that we spoke just below his hearing level, but we were only 12.

In many ways we were totally opposite. I was liberal and in liberal arts; he was conservative and in business. But Bob was the kind of person I could talk to once a year and feel as if we had just talked the night before. It was good to talk to someone who knew me from way back. He was shocked when I told him about my attack and he asked, "Now, I know you're going to be tough, but are you going to be smart tough or stupid tough?" I reassured him that I was being smart tough, and told him I was closing in on a 34-inch waist. We had both worked in some of the same stores while in college; if nothing else, we knew how to fold a pants leg under to pin it for a tailor and what size waist was appropriate for one's height. Our 20-year high school reunion was coming up and I wouldn't be able to get back to New York for it, so I asked Bob to send my regards and report back to me. He had one early sobering report; a guy from our junior high school class had died the year before of a cerebral hemorrhage at age 37. I guess I wasn't too young for a heart attack after all; we were at the age when mortality looks a lot more real.

At the end of the month, Jayne and I went to the fourth *Washington Star* reunion. The *Star* was Washington's afternoon paper that had gone out of business in August 1981. I was Religion Editor at the time—not "Religious Editor," as I was often introduced. I always explained that we had several religious editors, but they were in other departments. I caused a minor stir with news of my attack. One friend, Sheilah Kast, now with ABC News, asked if I were bitter about my attack because it came after I had lost weight and started exercising. I said I wasn't bitter because I figured that if what I had done had delayed my attack by just 12 hours, it had saved my life. If it had happened while I was in a bus stuck in traffic on I-95, I might well not be here right now.

The next major stage in my recovery was beginning my cardiac rehabilitation program. After my stress test, I talked to Sue Wingate, the nurse coordinator at NOVA-CAT, and she said I should start coming on Labor Day, September 5. I couldn't wait to get to the old gym at George Mason University, where NOVACAT met. I met first with Sue, who explained the program. She began by looking over a copy of the report on my stress test, and said, "This is average for a man your age who hasn't had a heart attack." That was what I wanted to hear—so much for being in good shape if I were 65.

The program worked like this: we met twice a week, Monday and Thursday, at about 5:00 P.M. We wore loose clothes and walking shoes; there was a locker room with a shower we could use if we wanted. We each had a card in a file box where we logged in the date and our weight. We had our blood pressure checked before we went to the gym. It wasn't air conditioned, but one side rolled up and was open to the outside air. For the first few visits, Sue hooked new patients up to a portable monitor—much like the little one I wore in the hospital, not the Holter—to keep track of their heart rates as they exercised.

We began with stretching exercises to loosen up our muscles and to reduce the risk of pulls and tears. Then we did some basic exercises—trunk twists, sit-ups, leg-raises, and so on. After the basic exercises, we began walking around the track. This was the warm-up period, which was important because it got our hearts pumping. If you begin exercising flat out without a warm-up, you can place too great a strain on your heart. The heart functions better as exercise progresses. I had noticed that, when I walked around the lake, my last lap was usually faster than my first. This explained why: the more I walked, the more efficient my heart became.

After the warm-up, we walked or jogged for 30 minutes. The recommended exercise level is 30 minutes of exercise that gets your pulse rate up to your target level three to five times a week. Less than three isn't enough; more than five increases the risk of injury. There was a boom box that played music for inspiration. (The music selection was fairly limited; I brought in a tape of *Hooked on Swing* to liven it up a little.) After the walking/jogging period, we "cooled down," walking a few more laps at a leisurely pace. Once a week we had a lecture on some aspect of cardiac care, such as exercise, nutrition, and so on.

The cooling-down period was as important as the warm-up because it allowed our heart rates to begin to lower from their exercise peaks. If you're exercising all out and your heart is pumping super-efficiently, and then you stop cold, your heart will continue to circulate blood at the same rate—for a brief time. What happens is that the blood leaves your head (and brain) expecting to be immediately replaced—except that it isn't replaced, because you're no longer exercising to circulate it back. The result is a sudden loss of blood in your brain—and a flat-out faint. Once you faint and lie down, the circulation returns to normal and you're fine. But it's something to be avoided.

The cooling-down period is important for another reason. If you go directly from peak exercise into a hot shower, while your blood is still circulating rapidly, the heat from the water will draw blood toward the skin and away from the heart. The result could be that the heart doesn't get the blood and oxygen it needs, and your blood pressure drops rapidly; you could even have a heart attack.

On my first day, I looked at and talked with the other people in the program to get a sense of where I fit in. The group was almost all men, but there were a few women. I was probably 10 years younger than anyone else in the room, and there were some guys in their 70s. Many had had bypasses, including some of the older men. It was something to watch those guys walking and jogging around the track; having some guy in his 70s who's had a triple bypass breeze past you is quite a lesson in what the heart can do. (One week I asked someone how he was doing. He said, "Not bad for an old guy with a heart attack." I said, "Hey! That's what I want to be when I grow up. I've already had a heart attack—now I just have to get to be an old guy.")

The two physicians who, along with Jim Metcalf, had founded NOVACAT—Cy Guynn and Robert Matthews —took turns coming to the program. They usually jogged along with everyone else and kept an eye on how the patients were doing. On my first night, Cy walked with me awhile and gave me the NOVACAT philosophy. He offered exactly the kind of sophisticated, nuanced, carefully worded medical advice I needed—"Screw the damaged part." That was history, he said, but the rest of my heart could do wonders, and that's what we were going to do. *That* was my kind of doctor.

Being in NOVACAT encouraged me to walk even more on my own. Two days later, I added a lap around the lake and was up to 4.2 miles a day. My third night at NOVACAT, though, I got a first-hand lesson in the importance of cooling down. Before we started, I chatted with Jim Metcalf, and he emphasized again the importance of cooling down. He explained again in detail what happens when the blood leaves your brain and doesn't come back. When we started walking, I got going at a pretty brisk pace. I was still on the monitor, and I was going over my training rate. Sue called me over to make sure I was OK, and I thought, "I'm stopping too quickly . . ." The next thing I knew, I was flat on my back on the grass just outside the gym and Sue was kneeling next to me holding the electric paddles on my chest in case she needed them. Luckily, she didn't. I had just been a text-book case of what happens when you stop exercising too quickly: the blood left my brain, I fainted and as soon as I was prone, the circulation returned to normal. When the blood hit my brain again, it was invigorating—it was like waking up after about 12 hours of the best sleep you've ever had, even though I was only out for a split second. I got up and started walking again, with Cy alongside and Sue watching the monitor, until we were all convinced that everything was all right.

The weekly lectures were a key part of the NOVACAT program. One week, Dr. Matthews discussed ventricular aneurisms, drawing one on the blackboard in the class-room where we met. After the lecture, I went up to him, pointed to his drawing and said, "I've got one of those." He said, "I've seen you walk. Forget about it."

By far the best-attended lecture was Cy Guynn's talk on sex and the heart. He asked how high we thought people's heart rates got during sex. Estimates were all over the place, including one of 160, made by someone who said he'd read an article on the subject. Guynn said, "Who were they studying? College kids?" He said a study of patients who had worn Holter monitors and had kept 24-hour diaries while wearing them found that the aver-age heart rate during sex was about 116 or 117, well within the "safe" limit. Based on my own experience with the Holter, however, I'd have to think the heart rate would get a little higher in someone not wearing a Holter. I couldn't figure out what to do with the damn thing when I had my pajamas on and had to brush my teeth, and I couldn't imagine what you'd do with it during sex.

Someone asked why, if sex were so safe, we were always seeing stories about men who died during sex. Dr. Guynn answered that most of those stories were about some guy in a motel with someone who wasn't his wife; it wasn't the sex that caused the heart attack—it was the anxiety. He said he had given that explanation a few years ago, and a man came up afterward and said, "Doc, I feel better now about sex with my wife, but you've got me worried about sex with my mistress." Guynn asked him how long he had been seeing his mistress, and the guy said four years. Guynn said he'd probably passed the point of peak anxiety by now and there wasn't any more risk in having sex with his mistress than with his wife.

One evening a few weeks after I started at NOVACAT, a new patient came in who was even younger than I, by a year or so. I tried to build some camaraderie with him, but I couldn't get through his bitterness. He was a marathon runner who had had a heart attack because of a spasm in an artery. The result was 25 percent damage to his heart. I told him that I didn't know exactly how much damage I had—"a lot" was as detailed as I wanted to hear; I just knew the damage was less than 40 percent, because a person can't live with 40 percent damage. I then told him that I'd probably be happy to have only 25 percent damage. I tried to tell him he'd be running again in no time. He didn't want to hear it, and he never came back.

When you're around cardiac patients, you hear a lot of stories—some encouraging, some scary. Here is one of the encouraging ones: a guy was having severe chest pains about five years after a bypass; the doctors did a new angiogram, found no new blockages, and blamed the pain on stress. Blockages often reoccur after a bypass, and he now had proof that he was all clear.

One night, two horror stories made the rounds. One

was about a guy who had chest pain, called his doctor to make an appointment for that afternoon, took a hot shower, and never came out. That certainly brought home the importance of cooling down after exercise and before a shower. Another was about a guy who had chest pains and waited while his wife put on makeup to take him to the hospital. He dropped dead in the emergency room; if she had gotten him there sooner, he'd probably still be alive. (That night, I told Jayne the story and said that I wanted to thank her for not stopping to put on makeup when I called her for help. "Makeup?" she said. "I wasn't even wearing underwear!")

NOVACAT was a source of good exercise tips. For example, when you're walking or running, it's important that your arms move back and forth, not right and left across your body. It's more efficient if they move back and forth; if they move across your body, they slow you down and make walking more difficult.

Jim Metcalf had some good tips about lifting. He talked about progressive weight lifting: starting small and adding a little weight at a time. He encouraged people to lift weights—after they got their doctor's OK—because the more muscle you had, the less strain there was on the heart when you did lift something.

Jim said that when you lift something, you should blow air out at the precise moment you lift; this reduces pressure and lowers the risk of a stroke. He also explained that shoveling snow was no problem if we treated it like exercise—pace yourself, check your heart rate, and don't overdo it. He told us to avoid what his mother used to call "a lazy man's load." That's a load that's too heavy because you're trying to make fewer trips. If you're shoveling snow, do one shovel's worth at a time; don't try to get half the driveway done at one time.

Because most of the other people at NOVACAT were jogging, I temporarily gave in to peer pressure and tried it myself. I could go along fine for a tenth of a mile or so, but then I ran out of breath. Sue ran with me one night to see what the problem was, and she said that the rest of my body hadn't caught up with my heart and wasn't in as good shape. I decided to give up jogging anyway. I'm pigeon-toed, and I figured that if I ran, it was only a matter of time until I kicked myself in one ankle with the other heel. That might do enough damage so that I couldn't even walk for a while. I had always admired Jackie Robinson; one reason I became a Dodger fan as a kid was that the Dodgers had broken the color line by hiring him. But I probably never admired him as much as when I tried running and realized that he'd been an incredible runner and base-stealer while being severely pigeon-toed. That's quite an accomplishment.

In addition to going to NOVACAT twice a week, I continued to walk on my own. By the middle of September, I was walking five miles three times a week. I spent so much time walking around the lake that I saw the same people and even some of the same neighborhood cats often enough to recognize them.

But I still had some unfinished business. One Sunday in late September, after walking five miles in the morning, I dragged Matt to the neighborhood basketball court in the afternoon and played a few games with him. Thanks to an unorthodox shot that was part hook and part heave that I had perfected when I was 12, I beat him. Of course, I was still taller than Matt then, and he wasn't exactly muscling his old man. But I had made my point to give him some reassurance—if I could beat him one-on-one after walking five miles, it was a good bet I wasn't going to drop dead any time soon.

Time was the best reassurance with the kids. They both watched me and said "Are you all right?" if I looked a little tired or distracted—they still do. One day I dozed off during a long car ride and Dan woke me up, saying, "I thought you were dead." But one day while we were having breakfast, he looked up and said, "Boy, that skim milk and that walking really work."

I was feeling my oats now. My resting pulse rate—the rate first thing in the morning—was down to 60, and that practically qualified as "athletic." Nothing made me angrier than hearing people ask if I were doing too much or pushing myself too hard. I wasn't. I felt two things very strongly. First, given the kind of sedentary lifestyle I'd led before, I was doing more now than ever, and there was no reason I couldn't work as before. Second, I knew that keeping my heart in good shape was the best thing I could do for myself, my best insurance. I was still scared that if I were ever to stop exercising, my heart would atrophy and I'd die.

I actually had some black humor about my situation. Someone said I was now less likely than other people to have any more heart problems because I was following doctor's orders and was being regularly monitored so they could take action at the first sign of trouble. I thought about it and said, "You know, when my time comes, it's probably not going to be my heart that gets me. It'll be something else. So if I ever come down with something really ugly, I'll just start eating steak and eggs three times a day."

I had an appointment for a checkup with Dr. Herron on October 18. He was late for it because he'd had an emergency at the hospital. A man could barely breathe; they'd done an angiogram and found that all three arteries registered 100 percent blockages—it was a miracle he was getting any circulation to his heart at all. The surgeons did a triple bypass and saved his life. I told Herron not to worry about being late—I'm sure he was late for a few appointments the day we met.

This was a routine checkup, and I got a pleasant surprise—I didn't need another EKG, which meant I didn't have to have my chest shaved again. I have a lot of hair on my chest and they usually have to shave it in several places to attach the leads for the EKG machine. I end up with irritated skin as each new hair stabs me while it grows back. One year when I went for a stress test, the regular nurse, Terry, let a new nurse shave me. The new nurse must have thought she was shaving her legs, because she took long, long strokes that removed half the hair on my chest. I was ready to kill her, and Terry promised not to let anyone else shave me again.

But there was no shaving during this visit. Herron checked me out and made no changes in my medication. He said, "If it's successful, leave it alone." He was very upbeat, and he said that I was doing very well. Referring to my stress test, he said, "We have to show people what they can do." I thought there was some question as to who was showing whom, but I let it go. I was just happy to be getting good reports.

In fact, as the fall wore on, it became clear that I wasn't the one in the family with the biggest health problem. Jayne's problems continued, and changes in hormone medication didn't help. Her doctor was trying to avoid a hysterectomy because she was so young, but nothing seemed to work.

I did see that my health had an impact on people. Many people were genuinely concerned; they asked questions and compared notes on diet or exercise. But other people—generally about my age—pulled back; they seemed threatened. Maybe the sight of someone their age who almost died shook them up; maybe they saw me as a pressure to make changes that they didn't want to make in their own lives. I don't know.

But I can't claim a perfect attitude myself. Twice I met women whose husbands had died of heart attacks, and I felt extremely awkward—and guilty. I suspected they felt awkward, too. How could a woman not feel uncomfortable around someone who had survived the same thing that killed her husband?

For the first six months after my attack, and even longer, Jayne told anyone with even a flicker of interest about what had happened to me and how I had recovered. She didn't do this because she wanted sympathy, but because she was proud of me. It reminded me of when Dr. Herron would look at me, look at my record, and shake his head ever so slightly, as if he still couldn't figure out what I was doing there. By the fall, Jayne had paid me the ultimate compliment—she started to complain when I left a coffee cup on the kitchen table and didn't put it in the sink, or when I trimmed my beard and mustache and didn't get all of the little hairs out of the bathroom sink. You get a free ride when people think you're at death's door; my getting complained at was a sure signal that Jayne had started to heal.

As the fall moved along, I was working more and more. It was during this time that I learned some important lessons. I felt tense and anxious if I consciously pressed to meet a deadline; being aware of a time crunch made me uncomfortable. But I found that if I concentrated on the work, not the time, I felt better and still met my deadlines. The biggest lesson was that just plain hard work was not a problem; I could work long hours if necessary and I might get exhausted, but a good night's sleep took care of it. Stress, on the other hand, was completely different—it was the gift that kept on giving. If I got myself into a stressed state, that feeling didn't go away in a hurry.

The hardest adjustment was probably learning to work nine to five Monday through Friday; I was used to always "being on," working evenings and parts of weekends. I'd been trying to get away from this before my attack, but it came a little easier now. If I had a particular deadline, or if several deadlines hit at the same time, I could work an evening or part of a weekend as long as I knew this extra work was limited. I could work *this* Saturday or *this* evening, but I avoided it on a steady basis. If I worked in the evening, I tried not to work the following weekend. That's still the way I work, and it's turned out well.

I had a difficult decision a few weeks before Christmas. I had just finished a history of the Campaign for Human Development and I was looking forward to a break. Then I got a call from *People* magazine. It was right after dozens of American servicemen had been killed in an airplane crash in Greenland as they took off to come home for the holidays. One of the widows wanted to talk; she had spoken to her husband on the phone just before the flight, and he had been crying because he said he knew it wasn't safe. Would I fly to Tennessee the next day to interview her? I'd have to file my story the day after that. It would have been an emotionally wrenching story to do; I'd managed to avoid that kind of story my whole career. But it would have meant a byline in *People* and extra money for the holidays. If the exact same call had come the year before, there's no question that I'd have been on the plane. But it wasn't a year before. I turned the assignment down. That "No" was one of the most liberating things I've ever done.

By early January, about seven months after my attack, things were getting back to normal. I'd been going to NOVACAT for five months, but it was becoming a logistical problem. When I went, Jayne came home from work, drove me to NOVACAT, drove home, and then came back to pick me up. I got a different ride sometimes, but it was becoming difficult. I was still walking for exercise and would continue walking. If I drove, I'd have continued with the program, but I decided that the time had come to stop going if it caused stress. It wasn't practical for me to continue, but I've stayed on the mailing list and stayed in touch. NOVACAT gave me exactly what I needed exactly when I needed it; there aren't too many things in life you can say that about.

As I look back, I realize that it was just about this time

that I stopped keeping a diary. I knew that being a heart patient is a lot like being an alcoholic—one is always recovering, never cured. But being a heart patient was no longer my primary identity; it was time to move on.

6

NORMALCY

The further away you get from a heart attack, the more you realize that returning to normal means walking a tightrope. On the one hand, you don't want to live every second thinking of yourself as a heart patient, because there's much more to your life than that. On the other hand, if you're not careful, returning to "normal" can mean resuming the same bad habits of diet, exercise, and attitude that helped you become a heart patient in the first place.

I was very conscious of walking that tightrope in the winter and spring of 1986, as I approached the first anniversary of my attack. I felt terrific, but I still took precautions. For example, I know that when a person eats, blood flows into the digestive system and away from the rest of the body, so I made sure not to place any strain on myself until an hour or two after a meal. (When we ate at Chi-Chis, our favorite Mexican restaurant, I'd climb the two long flights of stairs from the ground level before a meal; after, I'd take the elevator.) I didn't see any need to carry my nitroglycerin tablets with me all the time, but I took them with me when I was traveling away from home, when I exercised, or when it was extra cold out. I might jog for a bus, but I didn't try to go from 0 to 60 in a few seconds; I knew I needed to warm up before taxing myself.

At this point, Jayne's health problems were worse than mine, as her doctors tried a series of different medications to bring her menstrual bleeding under control. They were still saying that the shock of my heart attack had jolted her hormonal system and caused her problems. I didn't think that kind of jolt would still have an impact more than six months later, but all the talk about it gave me another dose of guilt to handle—not only had I almost died and caused my family so much pain by having a heart attack, I had also caused Jayne all the pain she was now going through.

I noticed that I was going through some subtle changes. I started glancing at the obituary page, something I never did before. I think that's something you do with age, anyway, as the people—entertainers, sports figures, politicians, scientists—who were part of your youth start to die off and you see a part of your own history fading away as well. I also saw how many people close to my own age hadn't been as lucky as I was. And I noticed that if I saw that so-and-so had died at, say, 73, I thought, "Too young." I'd become greedy for life; now that I'd had a close call, I wanted the whole nine yards, I wanted to get to be *really* old. I at least wanted to get what country singer Moe Bandy asked for—"Lord, don't let that cold wind blow till I'm too old to die young."

And as I read the papers and magazines and listened to the TV news, I realized that heart disease had become "my disease" in the same way that the Dodgers were "my baseball team." Just as I'd scan news of the Orioles or Yankees and read every word of every news story on the Dodgers, I found myself scanning news stories on other illnesses but devouring every word about new heart research. And hardly a month went by without some new study coming out. I realized that just as the world of cardiac care had changed dramatically in the five or ten years before my attack, it was changing at least as dramatically today. In line with heart disease being "my disease," I volunteered to collect for the American Heart Association in my neighborhood, and either Jayne or I have done it ever since.

I felt a bond with other heart patients, something like belonging to a secret club. I thought about that every time I heard an ambulance siren early in the morning. As a person sleeps, the body slows down production of the enzymes that fight blood clots, so most heart attacks occur in the morning. I know that not every early morning siren is responding to a heart attack, but I know that many are, and every time I hear one, I send a silent message of good luck to someone about to begin the adventure I went through.

I usually heard those sirens when I was walking to or from the lake, but as the weather grew colder, I could walk less often. I worried that my heart would suddenly get weak if I missed too much time, particularly if I'd had a cold or flu. But I was pleasantly surprised to find that if I went a few weeks or even a month or more without exercising, even though I might slow down a little, it only took a couple of days to get back to where I was before.

As my first anniversary approached, I thought it might be a good time to see about getting more life insurance. I called a salesman from the company where I already had a policy. His response was to press me to convert my term policy into whole life. Brilliant—just what I needed, to pay more money for the coverage I already had. I told him that right now I wasn't particularly worried about being able to afford the premiums on my old policy when I was 60; there was plenty of time to worry about that. I wanted to get some insurance for the next ten years, when my children would be growing up. I didn't expect to have another heart attack, but, God knows, I hadn't expected to have the one I had, either—and, of course, anybody can get hit by a truck. I filled out an application, got a physical, released my records from Dr. Herron, and waited to see what would happen. The insurance company didn't turn me down. When insurance companies don't particularly want to insure you, though, they "make you an offer" that they think will be too expensive for you to take; they were right. I didn't expect to get basic, cheap, nonsmoker rates, but what they asked was just too much at the time. I let Jayne call it. She said it was just too expensive, and she thought I should wait and try again in a few years. She reminded me that life insurance gets more affordable the further away you get from an attack, particularly at about five years. So I decided to wait.

I celebrated my thirty-ninth birthday on April 22, 1986, and it was the best ever. Forget "Life begins at 40"—this birthday was precious to me because I came so close to not seeing it. Jayne and I had very different attitudes as the next June 13 approached. She saw it as the anniversary of the day I had a terrible heart attack, and she was very uncomfortable. I saw it as the anniversary of the day I had a terrible heart attack and lived; I tended to see it as sort of a second birthday. When the day came, I walked up to the firehouse where the paramedics were based, but none of the people who had worked on me were there, so I left a greeting. I saved special food treats—like an Italian sausage and pepper sub or egg foo young—for special occasions like birthdays, my "anniversary," or good checkups.

Not long after, it was time for my annual treadmill test. This time, I did the same nine minutes, and my heart rate only went up to 170, not 180. That meant it was stronger than the year before; I could have gone beyond the nine minutes, but Dr. Herron said there was no point to it. I had done what I needed to do, and everything was fine.

By the summer of '86, Jayne's problems had worsened, and she finally decided to let her doctors perform a partial hysterectomy. She was only 36, and we had both heard plenty about doctors rushing into unnecessary hysterectomies, but this one hardly fit into that category. She had been weak and drained for a full year. A few years later, she had to fill out some medical forms that asked when her last period had begun; she wrote "June 13, 1985." The form asked how long it had lasted; she wrote "14 months." That was no exaggeration. She had the surgery in August. Some people she knew who had been through it said it takes about six months to fully recuperate. One day, they said, she'd wake up feeling terrific and wonder how she ever survived before. That was pretty much the case. After the doctors did a biopsy, they told her she had had about six different physical problems, and it was a miracle she hadn't bled to death. But now she had started to recover. And I got rid of a load of guilt; it certainly wasn't the shock of my heart attack that had caused all those problems. But we had both gone through a lot; Jayne kept saying, "How old are we really? Things are happening to us that aren't supposed to happen until we're in our 50s."

As the year went on, I became more aware that I was just drifting along, that too many things seemed out of my control. I didn't feel particularly creative at work, and I was losing some silly office politics games I shouldn't have lost. My relations with Jayne were getting strained, and I was always reacting to things, never acting, never taking charge. It took a long time for this awareness to bubble to the surface—with me, it usually does. But once it did, I realized what was happening. As my life had seemed to return to "normal" and I was less conscious of a day-to-day fight to recover, I had begun to feel less in control of my life. I saw that because of the suddenness of my heart attack, I had accepted a loss of control in my life as a given. Realizing what had happened didn't turn things around immediately, but it helped me turn the corner. I was surprised that my attack could cause this kind of reaction two years later, but I probably shouldn't have been—it was quite an attack and quite a shock to my body and mind.

I faced another bizarre aftershock that year. The brand-new mole that Jayne had noticed on my back when I came home from the hospital had grown rapidly and then stopped. I went to see my dermatologist, Dr. Kravitz, to have a small mole on my side removed, and he said, "I wouldn't mind seeing this one on your back come off, too." He said it was the size, color, texture, and in the location of the kind of mole that turns into one of the deadliest forms of skin cancer in men. He said he didn't think there was a problem now, but there could be one in a couple of years if I kept it. I let him take it off, and a biopsy found that he was exactly right. The mole had been benign, but there were active cells, and it most likely would have turned into cancer. I thought about how the mole appeared out of nowhere right after I had my heart attack and thought, "This is spooky"—my heart hadn't killed me one way, and now it was trying to do it another way. When Jayne went to see Dr. Kravitz about a skin rash awhile later, he told her she'd done a good job in catching the mole; he said I'd have been dead in five years. Jayne had saved my life again.

My checkups were still going well. I duplicated the previous year's treadmill performance and had my medication changed. First, Dr. Herron took me off the Persantine; studies had shown that aspirin alone was as effective as the aspirin-Persantine combination in preventing clots. Second, he cut my Isordil back from four a day to three a day, telling me to skip the one at bedtime; studies had found that the drug actually works better when you take it after leaving it out of your system for eight hours or so.

We went on a really relaxing vacation that year. We

started out by driving to Colonial Williamsburg, one of
our favorite places. Except this time. We spent about a
half hour going through the various shops and busi-
nesses and listening to lectures, and we all decided at
once that it was too much like school and work. We left
the colonial area and drove along a riverbank; we got out
and just sat, threw stones into the water, and generally relaxed. We were going to spend the rest of our vacation at
an old resort called the Chamberlain in Hampton, Virginia, and we added an extra day there. For the most
part, we sat by the saltwater pool and got some sun; the
service and food were great. All in all, it was the most
"nothing" I'd ever done. I'd go crazy doing it all the time,
but it was wonderful; it set our family a new standard for
relaxation.

The more time that went by, the more I learned about
what I could do. We decided to have part of our large
laundry room converted into an office because the one
I'd been using had become too small now that I worked at
home practically full time. We found a contractor who
would do the job at a good price during the last week of
December, a slow time for construction. But he told us on
a Friday that his workers would be there on Monday to
frame the room, so we had to get the laundry room
cleaned out in a hurry. We cleaned and carried for two
days straight; this was more lifting than I can ever remember doing. We got it done, and I had no problems
other than the muscle aches one would expect after
something like that. (Naturally, after the workers framed
the room, we didn't see them again for two weeks, which
we spent with furniture and boxes stacked up in the family room. The contractor kept referring to this as "a small
job," but we couldn't have had any more aggravation if
we'd had them build an addition onto the side of the
house.)

Just as I'd learned how much I could take physically, I
soon learned I could also handle being scared to death

and having my heart broken. One night I was watching TV in the family room. Dan came downstairs nibbling on a chicken leg, and, for no apparent reason, Willie attacked him. He wasn't playing; he growled, grabbed Dan's arm, and wouldn't let go—I had to struggle to pull him off. As soon as I did, he seemed to change back into his old self. He looked confused, as if he couldn't understand why Dan was crying, and he tried to lick him to make him feel better. Dan had serious bruises and scratches, and I shudder to think what would have happened if I hadn't been there. Willie had been aggressive a few times before, but it had been nothing like this. Once we got Dan taken care of, we talked to our vet, Willie's breeder, and a dog trainer. Their advice was unanimous —we could no longer keep Willie. If this had happened once, it could happen again, and there might not be anyone around to protect Dan. We had to make other arrangements for Willie, and it was the hardest thing I've ever done. Matt and Dan stayed home from school for two days and cried; Jayne and I weren't much better. But there had been no choice.

Several months later, Dan was taking a bath in the boys' bathroom, and, though I wasn't paying close attention, I suddenly had a feeling that the water had been running for a long time and I hadn't heard from Dan. I went in to make sure that he was all right. I couldn't see his head because it was behind the shower curtain, but the rest of his body was stretched out in the tub. In the nanosecond between the time I screamed his name and the time he said, "What?" I thought he had hit his head and drowned; he was just relaxing. It took a while for my heart to stop pounding after that. I thought about my scare and Willie and my weekend of basement cleaning, and I figured I must be in pretty good shape—no "bad heart."

Keeping my heart in good shape often depended on the weather. Washington is very wet year round, very cold in the winter, very hot and humid in the summer—

and it has a very short fall and spring. I was finding it harder and harder to do all the outside walking I wanted and needed to do, so I tried a different approach. A new health club had opened about a half mile away, so I joined to use its fitness room, primarily to use the treadmill. I'd walk for a half hour at about a four-mph pace at a slight incline. I missed the fresh air, but it was good exercise and it got my pulse rate in the 132–138 range, where it needed to be.

About three years after my heart attack, I went to a conference at the University of Virginia in Charlottesville for a few days. After lunch on the last day, I suddenly felt ill—my pulse was racing, my stomach was upset, and I felt hot and dizzy. At first I thought it was something I ate. They had a bunch of little sandwiches and I'd picked up what I thought was a ham sandwich. It turned out to be cold corned beef, but I ate it without realizing what it was. I rested for a while and someone from the conference staff gave me an Alka-Seltzer. I felt well enough to rejoin the discussion later in the afternoon. When the conference was over, I got a ride back with a friend and was home by dinnertime.

I was all right that night, but I had the same problem again the next day at lunch. I had decided to take some graduate courses at George Mason University, and Jayne was going to drive me over to get the forms after lunch. As we got to school, I felt as if I were having a monster anxiety attack. I'd been out of school for almost 20 years, but I wasn't particularly nervous about going back, so I was puzzled.

The symptoms went away after a while, but they came back the next morning after breakfast. I called Dr. Herron and he said it sounded as if I were having a reaction to the Procardia. I took it after meals and hadn't made the connection, thinking I was having a problem digesting my food. He prescribed another calcium channel blocker; he said this one did not normally produce the same reaction. But it did. I called that evening and spoke with the new partner in the practice, Dr. Pollock. He said to see what happened when I took a nitroglycerin pill and to come into the office first thing in the morning.

I took a nitroglycerin pill, and I felt pain racing through my chest. I wasn't going to take any chances; I called the paramedics again. I said I was sure it was a reaction to medication, but, with my history, I wanted to be sure. The paramedics took me to the emergency room at Fairfax Hospital. There, the doctors ran some tests and hooked me up to a heart monitor for a while until they were sure everything was OK.

I saw Dr. Pollock the next morning, and he said that, given the configuration of my arteries (with my very large left one), I would probably do as well without a calcium channel blocker as I had been doing with it before I developed a reaction. They had prescribed it to cut down on the chance of spasm in the artery before my angiogram. The angiogram had shown that there were no blockages in my healthy artery, so we knew that it was unlikely that a spasm could close it off. It was unusual to develop a reaction to a medication after almost three years, but it was not unheard of. Some people develop reactions to antibiotics as adults, and others outgrow allergies. As I shed yet another medication, I thought about the aspirin and the Lanoxin and joked that some day I'd come in and they'd take away all the pills and just tell me to chew some tree bark.

Dr. Pollock said I should have another stress test in a few days to make sure I was doing all right without the calcium channel blocker. When I took the stress test, I had my best one ever; in nine minutes, I only got my heart rate up to 154 and didn't even break a sweat. Walking had done wonders for me, and using the treadmill had improved upon that.

Even though I was fine, my reaction to the medication made me a bit more cautious for a while, and I decided to take a few precautions. People for the American Way was going to send some people to both political conventions that summer, and though they hadn't decided exactly who was going, I was a likely possibility. I thought about the heat and humidity of Atlanta in July and New Orleans in August, the long hours and fast food, and the highly charged atmosphere, and I said, "Who needs it?" I passed the word that I wanted to skip the trips.

If I sometimes felt older than my years, there was one benefit to being a baby boomer. Business was always looking to please my generation as a market, and my generation was now concerned about fat and cholesterol. With each passing month there were more healthful foods to choose from in the stores. As far as I'm concerned, the major breakthroughs came in the world of snacks. If you can eat Edy's Grand Light chocolate mousse ice cream with 120 calories, no cholesterol, and only four grams of fat in four ounces, life is good. If you crave a Hostess cupcake, they now make Hostess Lights—although I don't think they'll ever be able to come up with a "light" Twinkie.

Perhaps the greatest breakthrough was in my favorite sweets. When I was a kid in New York, I grew up eating Entenmann's coffee cakes, but I couldn't find that brand when I moved to Kansas City in the early seventies. Once when I went to Philadelphia for a weekend to cover a conference, I called a friend in New York and asked him to meet me for dinner. As a typical New Yorker who thought of Kansas City as a cultural wasteland, he asked if there were something he could bring me. The first thing I thought of was some Entenmann's coffee cake, particularly banana crunch. He brought me two cakes, and when I got home, I doled out little pieces to friends as though the cake were gold. A few years later, I was distraught when I heard that the company had gone out of business, but delighted when I later heard that Entenmann's had revived. When I was at National Catholic

News Service, somebody brought in a coffee cake, and people thought I was crazy for whooping and hollering when I saw it was Entenmann's. One day in early 1990, Jayne called to say she was just leaving the grocery store and told me to meet her in the driveway; she had a surprise. The surprise turned out to be Entenmann's Light, no-fat, no-cholesterol coffee cakes—and there was banana crunch. Jayne said people were fighting one another for the last boxes at the display.

My treadmill walking had improved my conditioning, but exercise became a problem the following winter and spring. I developed severe pain in my lower back and in my knees. One rainy Saturday, my knees hurt so much that I went to an urgent care facility to get them checked. I had X-rays taken, and the doctors didn't find anything wrong; they gave me pills for inflammation. But the pain didn't go away, and the pain in my back got worse.

It became clear that I had to do something, but I had heard many horror stories about people with back pain bouncing from doctor to doctor for years without any relief. All these stories made me reluctant to enter that game. Then I realized that if there were self-help books for heart patients, there were probably self-help books for people with back problems. I went to a nearby bookstore and found *Backache Relief* by a doctor, Arthur Klein, and a former *New York Times* reporter, Dava Sobel. The authors had done a survey of hundreds of people with chronic back pain to find out who or what had given them relief. Orthopedists were at the bottom of the list. Near the top were podiatrists. This seemed surprising at first, but I realized that it really made sense. My problems had begun after I had started walking seriously, and I suspected that the problems were coming from where the rubber met the road.

The book said one common problem that podiatrists found was a difference in leg lengths; just the slightest difference could lead to back strain. I went to see a nearby podiatrist, and he ruled out leg length as a problem for me. But it turned out that my flat feet were even flatter than I had thought. He prescribed "orthotics," shoe inserts made of space-age plastic that realign the feet and legs to relieve strain. He said that if I did a lot of walking with my condition, I'd experience incredible strain in my knees and lower back—exactly where I was feeling pain.

It took a few weeks to have the orthotics made, and during that time, I tried walking at a slower speed on the treadmill to reduce the strain. That helped, and when I got the orthotics, they helped as well. I can still overdo it, but the combination of slower speed and orthotics has been a great help.

Other strains were not as easy to deal with. After several years of working in a different way—primarily writing books and working with People for the American Way—I was feeling increasingly frustrated. At one level, I wasn't seeing my name in print often enough. That sounds crazy coming from someone who was still writing two weekly columns—George Gallup and I were now writing a weekly Gallup Religion Poll column—but it's the truth. Part of it was ego; I was used to seeing my name in print. Part of it was boredom. Even though I didn't want to go back to daily deadlines, I wanted to do more writing than I was doing; I felt I was going stale. One of the things I liked most about journalism was that I was always learning something new, and I felt that hadn't been happening lately. I also realized that I was a writer, not a politician. I was used to making my own decisions, going with what I had; I didn't think it should take eight people four drafts to write a four-paragraph letter. And my training told me that if nobody complains about what you're doing, you're doing a lousy job. I wasn't afraid of criticism, but most of the people I worked with were terrified of it.

I decided to do more free-lance writing, and I was

working on some things I thought would enable me to leave PFAW at the beginning of 1990. As is often the case, however, the decision was made for me. In July 1989, I became the victim of a "reorganization" that was the forerunner of a number of staff cuts to be made over the next few months. Leaving the place wasn't hard, but it was inconvenient. Though the job didn't provide all of my income, it provided a good chunk of it. It also provided my infrastructure—health insurance, pension plan, life insurance. I had to move quickly; the first thing I had to decide was what to do.

I'd been working more or less independently for almost eight years, and I decided it would be better to continue that way and add new clients than to try to jump back into the nine-to-five routine. I had to try to line up some regular clients, do some work to generate quick income, and replace my infrastructure. When the *Washington Star* had folded, I decided I wasn't going to rely on one source for all my income anymore; now I decided I wasn't going to put myself in a position in which I could lose my health insurance again. If getting life insurance after a heart attack is hard, getting health insurance on an individual basis after a heart attack is even harder. Luckily, the insurance world has responded to the growing number of people who work independently, and there were several group plans available. I joined the George Washington University program through a group plan for Washington Independent Writers, a professional organization for free-lancers. I also decided that it made sense to incorporate, so, in addition to everything else, I had to deal with lawyers and accountants and various bureaucracies on top of trying to line up business and trying to work.

The strain was mounting, and Jayne and I needed a break desperately. We immediately thought of the Chamberlain, the resort we had visited two years before. We made reservations for a few days in the middle of August. We knew Dan would be bored, so we hired a sitter to stay with him at home. (Our regular "sitter" wasn't available—Matt had joined the Navy after high school and was stationed in Japan, where he was off to a terrific start.)

On the day we were supposed to leave, the sitter had arrived, and Jayne and I were getting our things ready, five minutes from leaving, when the phone rang. It was my sister, Terri, calling from her office in New Carrollton, Maryland. She'd just gotten a phone call from the emergency room at Alexandria Hospital—our father had been found on the sidewalk, unconscious and bleeding from the head. That was all she knew. She said she was just leaving for the hospital. I called the emergency room, but the nurse I spoke to didn't know anything yet. It sounded as if Dad could have been mugged, but we immediately suspected that it had something to do with his heart.

Jayne and I drove to the hospital, and I thought about my father's heart problems over the past few years. He'd had a couple of bouts of congestive heart failure—this happens when the heart can't pump enough fluid out of the system. But these bouts had been brought under control with changes in medication. A couple of years earlier, Dad had needed prostate surgery, but the surgeon wouldn't operate unless he knew that my father's heart was stable. It wasn't surprising that Dad had never had an angiogram because they weren't given routinely when he'd had his heart attack in 1970. But, incredibly, he'd never had a stress test, either. His cardiologist gave him one and he didn't do well, so the doctor scheduled an angiogram. It showed that Dad had two arteries completely blocked and a 30 percent blockage—insignificant—in the third, with a lot of good collateral circulation. They said he should have no problem with the surgery, and he didn't.

When we got to the hospital, my father's cardiologist

was there, and he said the problem had been Dad's heart. But it wasn't another heart attack. Ever since his heart attack, my father had had an irregular heartbeat, an arrhythmia. Now he had had a serious arrhythmia, which had stopped his heart. He was unbelievably lucky to be alive now; he had been standing at a bus stop on the way to work when the arrhythmia hit. The doctors said he wouldn't have known a thing; he was unconscious before he hit the ground, landing flat on his face, breaking his nose and cracking his dentures. All this happened across the street from a firehouse—the paramedics there saw him fall, got to him immediately, and brought him to the hospital, which was only a few blocks away.

The doctors said they were concerned about possible brain damage because they didn't know how long his brain had been without oxygen, but they said he was strong to have survived so far and was showing early signs of regaining consciousness. Terri met us at the hospital, and we spent the day waiting for word. They said it was normal for someone in his condition to be unconscious for 24 to 48 hours.

Jayne and I stayed overnight at a hotel near the hospital and near my father and Terri's apartment. By the next day, Friday, the doctors were far more optimistic; they had not found any signs of brain damage, and my father was regaining consciousness. We saw him at noon, and he seemed to recognize us briefly. His doctors said it would take another couple of days for him to regain consciousness completely. There was nothing much we could do for a few days and we still needed some rest— now more than ever—but there was no way we could go to the Chamberlain, which was a six- or seven-hour drive. We decided to go instead to Annapolis, which was less than an hour away—close enough in case of another emergency.

We got to Annapolis in the late afternoon. We went to dinner and drove to the beach to walk around awhile.

When we got back to the hotel, I called Terri. She said Dad had had another arrhythmia, but the doctors had gotten it under control; he was doing fine. We spent much of the next few days on the phone with Terri, Dan, and the hospital. By Sunday night, I could talk to my father, who was having bursts of consciousness. We saw him Tuesday on the way back home just before he was moved to the Washington Hospital Center for tests. His doctors said the center was equipped to test him to see what was causing the arrhythmia so they could decide the best way to treat it. He had some short-term memory loss—he couldn't remember anything that had happened after he left the house on Thursday morning, and he kept asking where his dentures were and why his nose hurt, but he looked good, and he was even joking with his nurses.

I talked to him on the phone daily throughout the week, and Terri got to the hospital a couple of times. He sounded better every day, and though he didn't regain his memory, he understood what had happened. The doctors were supposed to do the tests on Friday, but he had a slight fever, so they postponed the tests until the following week. We all saw him on Saturday, and he really looked good. We brought him some yogurt and other foods he could eat without his dentures. We also brought him some things to read. Terri brought him an old transistor radio he'd had for years. Earlier, she had brought his calendar from home, and he showed us how he'd marked the days to keep track of where he was. On the day he'd gotten sick and the following days he'd written "lost," and on the next few days he'd written "half lost." He was in really good spirits. I told him a joke I'd just heard—"How do they give CPR in New York?" "Hey! Get up before you fuckin' die!"—and he laughed so hard I thought he was going to fall out of bed. Just before we left, he kissed Jayne and Terri, shook hands with Dan, and held my hand.

We talked again on Sunday. I called him about nine o'clock Monday night, and he was feeling good, laughing and joking. He wanted to hear the latest news from Matt in Japan and to hear what we were all doing. He had just talked to his brother Tommy, who was about to have surgery on his shoulder; he had broken his collarbone twice as a teenager, and it had given him trouble his whole life. Dad needed to hang up because Terri was trying to call, and the hospital was going to turn off the switchboard to the rooms soon. We were all still anxious to see how the tests would go so we would know what treatment they were going to use, but the doctors were all upbeat. I went to sleep thinking it was good to know he was doing so well.

I never heard the phone ring. The next thing I knew, it was 1:45 in the morning, the lights were on, and Jayne was on the phone. I heard her say, "Just say it, Terri. What happened?" A second later, she grabbed my hand and said, "Jim, your father's gone." He'd had another arrhythmia, and the doctors hadn't been able to control it. We couldn't believe it. I kept saying, "But I just talked to him," and I could still hear his voice in my right ear. Jayne told Terri to take a cab to our house, and I took a Valium while we waited; I was so shaken I could barely crawl out of bed.

When Terri got here, we were recovered enough to call the hospital. I finally reached the doctor who had been treating my father when he died. She assured me that he had received immediate attention, but his heart had just given out as they were working on him. Then, in that way doctors have of talking, she said, "You know, your father had a history of sudden death." Doctors use that term to describe the kind of arrhythmia my father had because sudden death is usually the result; he'd been so strong that it took three to kill him. But the language was bizarre—hearing about a "history of sudden death,"

I thought, "Yeah, when we were kids, we had to keep telling him 'Dad, cut that out—you're scaring Mom.'" But it wasn't a bizarre joke.

We somehow got through the night. The next morning, I told Dan what had happened; he ran into his room and didn't talk to anyone for hours. He and my father had been very close; Dan would call my father and Terri a couple of times a week to talk. Jayne called Matt in Japan. Phones are so scarce there that he never had one in his room, but we had his work number, and Jayne called and left a message. They reached him pretty quickly, and when we told him what had happened, he said, "I'll come home for the funeral." We'd always heard that the Navy takes care of its own, and it did. They gave him time off and coordinated with the Red Cross to get him on a plane home. He was going to meet us in New York; my mother's ashes are in a cemetery there, and my father had wanted to be interred next to her. When Dan heard that Matt was coming home, he talked for the first time.

That afternoon, Jayne drove Terri back home to pick up some things so she could stay with us until we left for New York on Friday. I asked Jayne to tell Terri to bring me my father's hairbrush. It was a weird request, but there was a reason for it. When I was in seventh grade and my friends and I all began "training" our hair— which in those days meant applying large gobs of Brylcreem or Vaseline Hair Tonic (or just plain Vaseline) and water—I had borrowed my father's hairbrush. It was a military-style brush, with a yellow handle, made by Fuller Brush. Being a fairly typical seventh grader, I'd misplaced it. My father seldom got angry, but he got angry when he couldn't find the brush; he said he'd had it since before he was married. I remember thinking, "What's the big deal about some old brush?" We finally found it; I think it turned up behind a radiator.

Over the years, I'd regularly see the brush soaking clean in the bathroom sink. As I got older, I came to appreciate how some things come to mean a great deal to you just because you've had them so long. Touching them is a link to your past. Every once in a while, when we were over at his place, I'd open the medicine chest just to make sure the brush was still there, and I'd smile when I saw it. No one else knew any of this, and I didn't want to take the chance that Terri would inadvertently throw out the 45-year-old brush. And then it hit me: my father never knew that story either, because I'd never told him. And then something else hit me: there was a story behind that hairbrush, and I'd never know what it was, because in the 30 years since I'd lost it behind a radiator, I'd never asked. You always think there's more time to do and say and ask; there isn't.

While Jayne and Terri were out, Jayne was worried about me and how my heart would handle the shock of my father's death. She called my doctor's office to ask if I should be doing anything—taking a mild tranquilizer, taking megavitamins, or doing something else. Without realizing it, she was looking for assurance as much as advice. As it happened, Dr. Herron was out and Dr. Marder took her call. Instead of reassurance, he gave her a lecture about how she shouldn't call a cardiologist about a psychiatric problem just as she shouldn't call a psychiatrist about a heart problem. He told her to tell me to call a psychiatrist and said, "We don't do stress management."

The next few days were rough as we went through the usual rituals and preparations. The hardest day was the day Jayne and I had to go to the funeral home to sign the death certificate. It was hard enough seeing his name— James Jacob Castelli—typed in, but the cause of death was a kicker. The immediate cause of death was arrhythmia, which stemmed from a ventricular aneurism from his heart attack 19 years before. The funeral attendant asked if I wanted to view the body. My first reaction was to say no, to avoid the pain. But Jayne urged me to see him. When her father had died in Florida, she almost didn't see his body because the coffin was closed at the funeral. She had made them open it so she could see her father; if she hadn't seen him, Jayne said, it would have been harder to accept his death. I gritted my teeth and we went in to see him. When we did, I started to laugh—if his color had looked like that in the hospital, we'd have said, "Looks good, looks good." He had never looked his age—he was 70—and I said, "God, dead he looks better than half the people who'll be at his funeral." But it would still be his funeral; we said our goodbyes and left.

One of my chores was to place his obituary. I didn't worry about the Washington paper; there was only one paper that counted, the *Mount Vernon Daily Argus*. He'd spent most of the first 62 years of his life in Mount Vernon, and he seemed to know everyone there; he couldn't walk a block without running into someone he knew. I gave the basic information to a woman in the obit department, and she kept asking for more information. He had been the superintendent in an apartment building in Mount Vernon for 17 years before he retired and moved to Virginia, but I knew that any obituary would be incomplete if it didn't mention his first love. He'd been a musician, a drummer, who'd played in local bands—from big bands to trios—for more than 20 years, and I made sure that information got in. When we got to New York, my aunts told me that they couldn't find my father's obit on the obituary page the day I'd been told it would be in. Then a neighbor called and said the newspaper had run it on page 3. I cried over that; that would have been the big time to Dad, and I was happy to see that the death of someone who wasn't famous, just a nice guy who knew everybody, was still "news."

When we were in New York, I saw aunts and uncles and cousins I hadn't seen in 15 to 20 years. As I talked with members of my father's generation, I realized that when people get to a certain age, they don't fear death, or, at least, there are things they fear much more. They don't want pain and suffering, and they don't want to live like a vegetable. My father was gone, but he'd been spared both of those fates. We'd been calling him "Mr. Lucky" because he'd fallen right across the street from the paramedics. He wasn't lucky enough to still be alive and well, but he'd died without pain after going to sleep happy after talking to his family. That's still a lot luckier than dying at a bus stop.

After the service, I told Dan I was proud of him for acting so grown up. He'd wanted to wear a sweater my father had given him the previous Christmas, even though the temperature outside was probably 80 degrees, and he'd just acted, well, grown up. Jayne said I wasn't doing him any favors by praising him for acting grown up because he was still a child, just short of 11; her point was well taken. But Dan had been strong and caring, and when I said he'd been grown up, he didn't know what I meant; he couldn't understand that there was any other way to behave. I was very proud of him. After we were back home, I told Matt how much it meant that he'd come back. I said we'd have understood if, given the time and distance and expense, he couldn't make it. "I know," he said, "but if I hadn't come, I just wouldn't have felt right. And I thought I'd be enough of a distraction that it would help everyone else." I was proud of him, too; when your child can say something like that, you know you've done something right.

After we all got home and Matt went back to Japan, I started to deal with the aftereffects of shock. Not surprisingly, my concerns focused on my heart. Rationally, I knew that my ventricular aneurism and my father's were quite different; he had had an irregular heartbeat from the day of his heart attack, and I had never had any. Emotionally, however, I knew no such thing. I started taking my pulse more often than usual, looking for problems.

To make matters worse, I came down with the flu, so I was feeling even weaker on top of all the stress. One day I felt weak and dizzy after climbing the stairs from our basement to the second floor. I took my pulse and felt what seemed like an enormous time between beats. I went to the emergency room and the doctors found no problems other than my being weak from the flu. The same sort of thing happened a week or so later. I called Dr. Herron on a Saturday morning and told him it felt as if my heart had skipped a beat. He said it was nothing to worry about and that I should be concerned only if I got dizzy when it happened. I was due for a checkup a couple of weeks after that; when Dr. Herron asked how I was feeling, I said, "Better than the last time I talked to you." My checkup was fine; I had survived a galloping case of cardiac neurosis.

All of this strain was taking a toll on both Jayne and me, and I felt as if I were close to exploding. On top of everything else, my Uncle Tommy had died unexpectedly from complications following his surgery, and that was an added shock. I had had enough of men with my face and last name dying. We desperately needed a break. I made a decision that, financially, wasn't the most prudent I've ever made but, psychologically, was one of the best— Jayne and I took a vacation in England and Scotland right after Thanksgiving. We had spent a week in London a few months before my heart attack, and it was the best time we ever had. Now we needed a break, but we wanted someplace familiar—this wasn't the time to learn a whole new culture. We got a sitter for Dan and left the end of November, arriving in London in time for Jayne's fortieth birthday. She's always loved the theater—she'd made a convert out of me—and I scored one of the great travel coups of all time: tickets to see *Phantom of the Opera* on her birthday and *Les Misérables* the next day. We saw a couple of other plays, revisited the British Museum, did some shopping, and enjoyed a bus tour to Edinburgh and surrounding areas. We had a great time, even if we did bring home the English flu that was sweeping the country—we were the first people we knew to have it after people like us brought it back to the states.

When we returned, I realized that I still had a long way to go when it came to working fun into my daily life. But I felt better knowing that I had learned that a dramatic break, like this trip, was necessary for survival. Taking time off and getting a change of scenery wasn't a magic solution—it didn't make life's problems go away. But when we got back, I was refreshed enough to deal with them again.

7

How Type A
Almost Killed
Me—And Then
Saved My Life

As my recovery continued, one of the things that still troubled me was the whole question of the "Type A" personality. I had no doubt that stress had played a major role in setting up my heart attack. But I was still uncomfortable with the stark distinction between Type A and Type B personalities. This distinction reminded me of an old joke: There are two kinds of people in the world, those who divide the world into two kinds of people, and those who don't.

I heard a great "Type A" story from Wes Pippert, a former reporter with UPI. While assigned to Israel, he had taken part in a test of U.S. embassy employees to diagnose Type A behavior. Each participant was given a long questionnaire to fill out by answering "always," "sometimes," and "never." The subjects were told to avoid "sometimes" answers as often as possible. Wes says that's what he did, even though he would have preferred to answer "sometimes" a lot more often. When the tests were scored, he came out a Type A. Wes said, "I talked to the people who came out Type B and found out they gave a lot of 'sometimes' answers. I said, 'They told us not to do that.' And the Type Bs said, 'Yeah, I know, but . . .' "

I guess I could see Type A and Type B as something like political parties, the Democrats and Republicans of life, but not as the only two personality types in the world. I knew some of my habits were bad for me, but I wasn't so sure about others. I thought being punctual was just a sign of courtesy if it weren't obsessive, and I still didn't see anything wrong with hard work and, yes, even being ambitious and a little competitive.

The first sign I had that I might be on to something was in an article entitled "The Hostile Heart" in the September 1986 issue of *Psychology Today*. "Type A research is now undergoing a change of direction," the article said, "and 10 years hence we may not be using the term at all."

It seems researchers had realized that the Type A personality demonstrated a mixture of behaviors and that some were "toxic" and some were not. The leader in this new research was Dr. Redford Williams at the Duke University Medical Center. Williams had found that the degree of hostility, particularly what he called a "cynical contempt," was even better than an overall Type A personality at predicting the amount of blockages in patients' arteries. He also found that patients expressing cynical contempt, a constant distrusting of others, were more likely than others to die from heart attacks and other causes.

Psychology Today returned to the subject just a few months later with a cover story, "Type A on Trial." This article began with a different approach; it reported that a number of major heart studies, including the famous Multiple Risk Factor Intervention Trial (MR. FIT) had failed to show that Type A personalities were more likely than others to have heart disease. Much of the article focused on arguments among researchers about the proper questions and technique to use to identify Type As. But it also went in more depth into research on the hostility component of Type A personality. Researchers saw hostility and repressed anger as key traits that lead to heart attacks. The article, by Joshua Fischman, said, "Studies have shown that hostile, angry people tend to be 'hot reactors,' who have very intense physiological reactions to stress."

Another researcher, psychologist Larry Scherwitz, concluded that self-involvement was a factor, and that people who say "I," "me," and "my" a lot are more likely to have heart attacks. He said, "Self-involvement leads to a feeling of isolation and incompleteness, promoting Type A behavior, hostility, and the incapacity to give and receive social support."

In January 1989, Williams published a new study concluding that angry, cynical people are five times likelier to die under age 50 than those who are trusting and calm. He said, "We can now state with some confidence that of all the aspects originally described as making up the global Type A pattern, only those related to hostility and anger are really coronary prone. . . . There is no evidence that Type A personality, meaning the workaholic, competitive, job-involved person, is predictive of premature death. But there is lots of evidence that hostility and anger are predictive."

Williams based his findings on a number of studies, including one of 118 lawyers over a 25-year period. Those who scored high on hostility on a standardized personality test taken in law school were five times likelier to die before age 50 than their non-hostile classmates.

Williams said personality traits such as paranoia ("People out there are picking on me"), social avoidance ("I'd rather cross the street than meet that person"), and neurotic behaviors did not correlate with early death.

But, he said, cynical mistrust ("People lie to get ahead"), anger, and acting out anger ("I often have to get rough with people") did.

Although many people get annoyed when, for example, they're on the express line at the supermarket and the person ahead of them has too many items, the angry personality type will act out his or her anger. Williams said angry people report more hassles during the day.

But Williams also said that this predisposition to anger can be biological. He said hostile people have a weak parasympathetic nervous system, which normally calms people down. Those with such systems produce adrenalin quickly and stay angry longer. They also have sharper increases in blood pressure than those with stronger parasympathetic nervous systems.

Williams later told *U.S. News & World Report* that "30 to 50 percent of the behavior pattern is rooted in the genes. But the way children are reared has a lot to do with whether that pattern will dominate in later life. Children who don't get unconditional parental love and care and lots of physical contact are more likely to be mistrusting, easy-to-anger adults."

In addition, Williams said, it's possible for angry people to change their ways: "Control your thoughts. If cynical, mistrusting thoughts cause you a lot of stress, you need to stop having them. When you start thinking, 'How inconsiderate of that woman not to have her check filled out when she gets to the head of the line,' become aware of that thought and sternly tell yourself to stop. You might also want to keep a hostility log, writing down every time you have those thoughts. Trusting other people to make some decisions for you can help you overcome the feeling that others are out to get you. Finally, though it sounds trite, try to enjoy life more. You only have a relatively short stay in this world, so why go around being angry all the time?"

Cardiologist Meyer Friedman, one of the two researchers who first came up with the notion of the Type A personality, hasn't given up on it yet. But his language today sounds a lot like Williams's. In the April 1989 *Psychology Today*, he said Type As suffer from the absence of a "spiritual life." Friedman said that by "spiritual" he didn't mean religious beliefs, but a "basic concern with human relations and other interests that enrich life."

But hostility and lack of a "spiritual life" may not be the only toxic components of the Type A personality. The October 1989 *Psychology Today* contained an article by psychologist Robert Levine on the relationship between the "pace of life" and coronary heart disease. Levine's researchers measured time urgency, the desire to make every second count, in a number of different-sized cities in different parts of the country. They found that the fastest-paced cities had the highest rates of coronary heart disease, and they concluded that time urgency contributes to heart disease.

But Levine said other researchers, including Jonathan Freedman and Donald Edwards of the University of Toronto, had found that time pressure is not always stressful and damaging; it can also be challenging and energizing.

"For individuals," Levine said, "the relationship between pace of life, personality, and CHD [coronary heart disease] isn't a simple one. Just as Type A settings may be stressful to Type Bs, Type As may experience distress when their surroundings are too relaxed for their tastes. The key is knowing one's limits and preferences. A good fit between our inner and outer worlds is a better predictor of health than any mailing address."

Finally, there's great irony in all the research on Type As. In January 1988, researcher David Ragland at the University of California at Berkeley released a study that defied the conventional wisdom. He found that Type As were actually twice as likely to survive a heart attack as Type Bs.

What do I, as a reformed Type A personality, make of all of this?

First, as one who has experience with both having a heart attack and recovering from one ("surviving" was out of my hands), I'm convinced that there is no contradiction here: Type A behavior—at least some of it— almost killed me, but it also helped save my life.

I'm convinced that being a Type A personality—and the stress it produced—was a contributing factor to my heart attack. I had many of the classic symptoms: I ate and moved quickly, I was impatient with the pace of life (long lines drove me crazy), I felt that there was never enough time to do what I had to do, and I felt guilty when I wasn't working. My career was in journalism, which, with its emphasis on competition and deadlines, and the practical necessity of doing at least three things at once, rewards, if not creates, Type A behavior. And, although I didn't smoke, as many Type As do, I was a caffeine addict.

But looking back, I see that I was also angry much of the time, often without knowing why or at what. Sorting it out, I'd say that anger and time urgency—either too much or the wrong kind—were important factors in producing the stress that contributed to my attack. They were more important factors than being ambitious or wanting to do a good job.

As for recovery, Ragland and others speculate that because Type As are more compulsive about taking their medication and following doctors' instructions, they have a better survival rate. That's not it. When I finally realized that I was having a heart attack, my first instinct was to fight back—something like, "Hell, no, we won't go." To the degree that I was conscious in the first hours, and as I began my recovery, that was my mood. That may be "aggression," and it may be "competitiveness," but what it came down to was fighting for my life, and not passively bemoaning my fate. If that makes me a Type A, so be it.

As I recovered, I discovered that my body was turning into one big biofeedback machine, sending me vital information about the impact of my behavior on my health. Put simply, if something made my chest muscles tense, it was bad for me; if it made them relax, it was good for me. So, for example, I found that exercise—even working up the kind of sweat that used to frighten me—was good for me. So was rest. So was having fun. I also learned that some things—like overeating or drinking caffeine— were bad for me.

This "biofeedback" approach also worked with Type A characteristics. Some Type A behavior is good for me. I found that plain old-fashioned hard work, even with long hours, felt good as long as it was satisfying. I'm still "ambitious" in the sense that I want to do a good job and get ahead. And there's nothing wrong with being on time for appointments if it's done out of courtesy and not compulsion.

But I also learned quite quickly that some Type A behavior was bad for me—and that stress, particularly avoidable stress, was the worst. I've always distrusted "born-again" experiences, whether in religion, politics, or lifestyle, and I guarded against a radical conversion that wouldn't last. But I have changed. I've learned not to panic at the sight of a long line at the bank or the supermarket. I've learned that it's not hard to turn down work projects that are guaranteed to produce more stress than they're worth. Before my heart attack, I never exercised or did anything with my hands (besides type), but I had by now learned to enjoy exercise. While I was recuperating, I started experimenting with cooking low-fat, low-cholesterol meals and found that I enjoyed it. Now, if I go too long without a good walk or cooking something for fun, I miss it—and I get back to it.

My "biofeedback" approach also showed me that hostility wastes energy and causes stress. One form this takes is that I'm much less likely to let things fester; I'm more likely to let people know when I think they're doing an inadequate job or wasting my time—and, now that I've been given "extra" time, I regard wasting it as an unforgivable sin. The research on the "pace of life" also fits; I don't have to feel guilty about being sensitive to the difference between being relaxed and being bored. But my therapeutic directness has also sensitized me to how much I appreciate positive relationships and experiences. To use a mundane example, when I eat out, I'm more likely to complain when the food or service is poor—and more likely to say thank you and tip generously when it's good. Overall, I'm considerably less hostile, and, possibly, even a little nicer since my heart attack.

The new research on Type A personalities has confirmed and legitimized my own experience; I now feel comfortable about getting rid of the parts of my personality that were destructive while holding on to others that are the best of me.

When I had my heart attack, I spent four days in the cardiac intensive care unit; I didn't even put my glasses on for the whole time, and I can barely see without them. But I kept my watch on. My doctors told me there are important plateaus that, when reached, indicate greater chances of survival—first 4 hours, then 24, then 48, then 96. I figured that if time were so important, I was going to watch it myself.

To this day, I won't take my watch off. But it's not because I still suffer from Type A "hurry sickness"—my watch is a reminder that all our time is limited. I don't want time to hurry past anymore; I want it to linger so I can enjoy it.

8

"THE CHOLESTEROL MYTH" MYTH

"The Cholesterol Myth," screamed the headline of the September 1989 *Atlantic Monthly*—"Diet has hardly any effect on your cholesterol level; the drugs that can lower it often have serious side effects; and there is no evidence that lowering your cholesterol will lengthen your life."

That was the opening salvo in an attack on the "heart establishment" launched by Thomas J. Moore, 45, an investigative journalist. The *Atlantic* article was an excerpt from his book, *Heart Failure*, published by Random House.

It was quite a grabber, and, like many other people with heart disease or high cholesterol, I read it avidly. It appeared at a time when my own cholesterol level was becoming of increasing concern. Over the four years since my heart attack, my weight had crept back up, and, with it, my cholesterol level. When I weighed 167 pounds, my cholesterol level was 189; when I weighed 178, it was 218; when I weighed 198, it was 241 and then 256. Also, my ratio of total cholesterol to HDL was dangerous; at one point, it was as high as 9 to 1, and now it was about 7 to 1. The goal is 4.5 to 1.

Dr. Herron wanted to put me on lovastatin, the newest cholesterol-lowering drug on the market, but I was resisting. I wanted to try to lower my cholesterol again with diet and exercise. I wasn't eating badly, but I learned that one can put on weight and increase cholesterol even by eating too much healthful food. I could eat pasta instead of roast beef, but I was still eating too much pasta. And though I was still exercising regularly, I wasn't walking 25 miles a week. Apparently my metabolism needs quite a bit of exercise to shake it up. I knew I wasn't going to let my cholesterol remain where it was indefinitely, but I also knew that, with no blockages in my healthy artery, another six months without lovastatin wasn't going to hurt me.

So I saw the *Atlantic* article as interesting both personally and professionally. I hadn't done anything for *People* for a while, and I thought the dispute between Moore and the heart establishment made a perfect story for it. I called the Washington Bureau with the idea at the same time that the New York office suggested the same idea, so I got the assignment to work on the story.

The fight was a good one. Not surprisingly, the heart establishment struck back, and the rhetoric was heated on both sides. Moore wrote scornfully of a small clique of cholesterol researchers in league to make millions for the drug companies by pushing dangerous cholesterol drugs. His critics responded by calling him irresponsible and charging that he would lead people with high cholesterol to skip treatment they badly needed.

When all the rhetoric was stripped away—and there was a lot of it—Moore and the heart establishment were not all that far apart. Leading heart researchers agreed with Moore that much more needed to be learned about the role of cholesterol in heart disease—particularly in women and the elderly—and that cholesterol-lowering drugs must be used very carefully. Moore conceded that

the link between cholesterol and heart disease is "strong-
est and most unmistakable in young and middle-aged
men"—the group most at risk of premature heart disease
and death.

And Moore, who said his cholesterol level is "about average," conceded that he follows a program of diet and
exercise not unlike the American Heart Association's
moderate plan. The difference, he said, is that he follows
his program because it makes sense to him, not because
he was ordered to do so by a doctor—or by his nemesis,
the National Cholesterol Education Program (NCEP)
launched in 1987 by the National Heart, Lung, and
Blood Institute. Moore said he objected to the National
Cholesterol Education Program on public policy
grounds—he saw the program as too much money chas-
ing too little cure.

The NCEP set a national goal of a 10 percent drop in
the nation's average cholesterol level, which is 215; the
program says this would result in a 20 percent decrease in
the death rate from coronary heart disease. Moore estimated that this would cost Americans $10 to $20 billion
a year.

These are the recommendations of the National Cholesterol Education Program:

- Everyone age 20 and up should have their cholesterol checked. If the level is below 200, test again
  every five years. If it's over 200, test again and use
  the average as a base for comparison; if the average
  is 200–239, retest yearly.

- People with cholesterol levels over 240 or those with
  200–239 who have either heart disease or one other
  risk factor should have a lipid profile, which shows
  the LDL and HDL counts.

- People with LDL of 160 or people with LDL of 130–
  159 and heart disease or two risk factors for it should
  go on a cholesterol-lowering diet.

- People with LDL of 190 or more, or people with
  LDL of 160 or higher and heart disease or two risk
  factors for it, who have not lowered their cholesterol
  after six months of diet, should use cholesterol-
  lowering drugs.

Moore, who lives on Capitol Hill with his wife, Barbara,
got into the cholesterol debate through the back door. He
began focusing on heart issues when he wrote a prize-
winning series on unnecessary and dangerous bypass
surgery for the Knight-Ridder newspaper chain. He is
now a visiting fellow at the Graduate Institute at George
Washington University. The research on bypass surgery
led to his current book. While traveling with Emergency
Medical Services teams trained to treat heart attacks on
the spot, Moore says, "I saw a lot of people die of heart attacks in front of my eyes. I wanted to do something on
prevention—that's why I looked at cholesterol. I expected to come up with a different story."

What he found, he said, is that the role of cholesterol
was being hotly debated in medical journals. He felt the
public was being given only one side of that debate.
Moore, who worked on Gary Hart's senate staff and was
an investigator into the CIA for the Senate Select Committee on Intelligence, approaches the cholesterol debate
as an issue of "information policy" from a leftist political
perspective that sees CIA-style conspiracies in the medical community.

He nicely demolished a straw man, arguing, "We aren't
anywhere near making cholesterol the sole cause of heart
disease"—although it's hard to find anyone who says it
is. Actually, Dr. Daniel Steinberg, professor of medicine
and director for the special center for research on ar-
teriosclerosis at the University of California at San Diego,
told me he would guess that cholesterol is responsible for
about half of the heart disease in the country. Steinberg
chaired a 1984 conference that targeted cholesterol as a

main cause of heart disease—a conference Moore criticized.

Scientists have debated the relationship of cholesterol to heart disease for decades, but within the past decade, the number of studies showing a positive relationship has grown. Moore argues that some of these results have been overstated, while his critics claim he ignored other significant studies. Moore counters that no author can cite every study.

But one major disagreement between Moore and the heart establishment involves interpretation of a simple chart that reflects the findings of the Multiple Risk Factor Intervention Trial (MR. FIT), a study of 361,662 men over a seven-year period:

Serum-Cholesterol Level	Living	Dead from All Causes	Dead from Heart Disease
Low (202 mg/dl or less)	97.8%	2.2%	0.5%
Average (203–244 mg/dl)	97.3%	2.7%	0.9%
High (245 mg/dl or more)	96.2%	3.8%	1.7%

The NCEP and the American Heart Association describe the results as showing that those with cholesterol 245 and above have three times the death rate due to heart disease as those with levels at or below 202—1.7 percent versus 0.5 percent. Moore argues that the absolute difference of 1.2 percent is much more modest than that—"You can look at it any way you want." I know I looked at it a long time, and, given a choice, I'd certainly prefer a low cholesterol level to a high one; I suspect most people will agree.

Moore also argued that lowering cholesterol does not

lower overall mortality—if fewer people die of heart disease, more die of something else. A number of scientists have made this point as well. But Dr. James Cleeman, coordinator for the NCEP, argues that "You can't estimate the benefit of cholesterol lowering on the basis of a five-year test; it takes a lifetime."

Dr. John LaRosa, dean of clinical studies and director of the lipid laboratory at George Washington University, said Moore had ignored evidence from cross-cultural studies. He said that the Japanese have average cholesterol of 160 and lower heart disease than Americans even though they smoke more and have higher blood pressure. "If a Japanese man goes to Hawaii, his cholesterol level goes up 15 percent and his risk of coronary artery disease goes up," LaRosa said. "If the same man goes to California, his cholesterol level and risk are indistinguishable from those of American men."

One subject on which Moore and his critics agreed is that because most research on cholesterol has involved young and middle-aged men, not as much is known about the link between cholesterol and heart disease in women and the elderly. The National Heart, Lung, and Blood Institute has begun a major study of cholesterol in these groups. Moore called this "A major, major step forward—that is a great study. The only problem is that it may try to answer too many questions at once and be hard to sort out. But the most important unanswered question is what happens with a dramatic change in cholesterol levels, and now they're going to try to answer it."

The principal dispute between Moore and the heart establishment involved the possibility of reducing cholesterol levels with diet. But even here, the difference turns out not to be great. Dr. Myron Weisfeld, president of the American Heart Association and director of the cardiology division at Johns Hopkins University in Baltimore, said that people can lower their cholesterol levels with diet by an average of 8 to 10 percent. Moore argued that studies actually show the figure is 5 to 7 percent—and, he argued, "It doesn't justify a national program to make a 5 percent change."

Again, Moore's critics disagreed. They argued that even a 5 percent reduction in cholesterol levels would translate into a 10 percent reduction in risk of coronary artery disease. Cleeman dismisses Moore's claim that the National Cholesterol Education Program will cost Americans $10–20 billion: "The percentage of people who need to be on drugs is very small, and a low-cholesterol diet costs no more than what they're eating now."

Weisfeld argued that Moore focuses too much on the small differences in the number of cardiac deaths found in some studies and pays insufficient attention to the findings on a lower number of non-fatal heart attacks among those who have lowered their cholesterol. Weisfeld said, "Cardiac disability takes much more of an economic toll on the country than testing cholesterol." Steinberg said, "If you prevent somebody's heart attack, you give him a lot of good years."

Weisfeld also noted that some people respond better to diet than others and can have large reductions in cholesterol level. For example, *Washington Post* columnist Bob Levy wrote that he had lowered his cholesterol from the 280s to the 190s in 13 weeks with diet and medication. Weisfeld said, "You can even actually reduce the level of plaque in an individual with diet."

Moore said that, like diet, drugs make only moderate changes in lowering cholesterol and, unlike diet, have unpleasant side effects and may be dangerous. The NCEP recommends the use of drugs for those with an LDL level of 190 (which translates into total cholesterol of about 265) who have not been able to lower their levels after six months of dieting.

Moore was especially critical of lovastatin, a new cholesterol-lowering drug with fewer side effects than cholestyramine, known for creating gastric problems. He argued that FDA approval of lovastatin was premature because not enough is known about its long-term effects. He also said one test suggested that lovastatin might actually cause heart attacks—a charge his critics deny.

Moore drew support for his criticism of cholesterol-lowering drugs from Dr. Allen Brett of New England Deaconess Hospital, who wrote about the subject for the *New England Journal of Medicine*. Brett argued that there is a greater burden of responsibility on doctors who prescribe medication than on those who prescribe diet because changes in diet are harmless, while drugs may cause harm. Even Brett, however, said, "Certainly, for patients with extremely elevated levels of cholesterol and multiple risk factors, the decisions may be relatively straightforward: there is more to gain if treatment proves beneficial and less to lose if the benefits are overestimated."

But, again, the differences here are less than meet the eye. Steinberg, Cleeman, LaRosa, and Weisfeld all warn of the dangers of overmedication. They point out that lovastatin is not the drug of first choice because not enough is known about its long-term effects; cholestyramine, Niacin, and Lopid are recommended.

Weisfeld also noted that physicians must still consider individual patients' situations when applying the guidelines. He says, "You have to consider family history, other risk factors, the relative level of cholesterol and age and stage in life. You could have two men with cholesterol levels of 250 to 260. One is 40 years old and has a father who died of a heart attack at 35 and a brother who's had two heart attacks at 45; I would find it possible as a physician to conclude that drugs would be in his best interest. You could have a second man who's 50, his father is 85 and his siblings are OK and he has no other risk factors. I'd be reticent to prescribe drugs because he's at far less risk."

Moore made the rounds of radio and TV talk shows,

often debating with medical experts. He said he learned two things from his experience. "The big surprise," he said, "is that there certainly are a lot of people out there. I'm amazed at the number of people who are willing to make really draconian changes in their diets to lower their cholesterol, who personally attribute to it a very important improvement in their lives. That's been the big surprise."

Another surprise: "One thing that has come out in my call-in shows is people who are undergoing great privation on cholesterol-lowering diets when the evidence for the elderly is so weak. People have told me about their mothers calling them in tears because they can't get enough to eat on the diets that they've been put on. Very serious, tragic stories, and I sense if you want a coming together that the elderly don't belong in this program."

The heart establishment marshaled its forces and mounted a major counterattack in November at the annual scientific meeting of the American Heart Association in New Orleans. First, the American Heart Association (AHA) and the National Heart, Blood, and Lung Institute issued a detailed joint statement calling evidence of the link between cholesterol and heart disease "overwhelming."

The statement said, "Epidemiologic, clinical, genetic, and laboratory animal studies all indicate that high plasma levels of cholesterol are causally related to atherosclerosis and to an increased risk of coronary heart disease. Clinical studies have shown that cholesterol modification by diet or drugs can lower that risk."

The 18-page statement summarized dozens of large-scale studies showing the connection between cholesterol and heart disease. It cited the following items:

- Four studies showing that groups with the highest level of cholesterol had the highest level of heart attacks and heart-related deaths.

- Three studies in which groups who reduced their cholesterol levels also reduced their heart attack rate.

- Seven studies showing that people with high-fat diets had higher cholesterol levels and higher heart-related deaths than those with low-fat diets.

- Animal experiments in which high-cholesterol diets produced rapid clogging of the arteries. The statement said that even though most of these studies were of middle-aged men, the two groups believed their findings also applied to women, the elderly, and the young. The AHA meeting also released three new studies showing that people who lower their cholesterol through diet or drugs can actually begin to clean out blocked arteries:

- Dr. Greg Brown of the University of Washington put people on two combinations of cholesterol-lowering drugs. Over five years, the fatty buildups shrank in 35 percent and got bigger in 23 percent.

- Dr. David Blankenhorn and colleagues from the University of Southern California also found a significant slowing of the disease in people treated for four years with cholesterol medicine.

- Dr. Dean Ornish of the University of California, San Francisco, put subjects on strict vegetarian diets and had them participate in exercise and relaxation programs. After one year, 82 percent showed overall regression of artery deposits.

Although these and many other studies were conducted on people at the highest risk of heart trouble, the doctors contended that sensible eating and lower cholesterol are good for everyone. Dr. Scott M. Grundy of the University of Texas in Dallas said, "Not only does diet make a difference, it is the major approach to cholesterol lowering across the board."

Other studies that have appeared since Moore's article lend further support to the heart establishment:

- A University of Pittsburgh study found that menopause appears to increase the risk of heart disease for women by causing harmful changes in their cholesterol levels. "As women go through menopause, they should have their lipids checked and if they see a change consider a number of options," according to Karen Matthews, a professor of psychiatry at the University of Pittsburgh, who headed the study.

  The study was the first to directly measure cholesterol levels in women before and after they went through menopause and compare the levels to other women in the same age group. The researchers tested 541 healthy women before they went through menopause in 1983 and 1984 for a variety of factors believed associated with an increased risk for heart disease.

  When the researchers compared the 69 women who went through menopause in the next two and a half years to women who did not, the women who went through menopause had about twice the increase in their blood levels' LDLs. The women who went through menopause also had a significant drop in their HDL levels.

  In addition, the cholesterol levels of 32 of the women who went through menopause but began taking supplemental estrogen did not change significantly, the researchers found. The use of estrogen by postmenopausal women remains controversial because it may increase the risk of cancer, Matthews said.

- A study conducted at Kuakini Medical Center in Honolulu found that elderly men with high cholesterol levels face an increased risk of heart disease.

The study of 1,480 men over 65 found that those with high cholesterol levels faced a 60 to 70 percent greater risk of heart attack than those with low cholesterol levels. Those with cholesterol levels over 250 were more than twice as likely to develop heart disease as those with levels under 200. The study was the second to show a relationship between cholesterol and heart disease in the elderly; the Framingham, Massachusetts, heart study had indicated similar results three years earlier.

• Officials of the U.S. Centers for Disease Control said cholesterol tests in adults as young as 20 can be used to predict who is apt to have dangerously high cholesterol later in life. The tests could enable people to change their diets or begin exercise programs before serum cholesterol levels get too high.

The researchers studied statistics on how cholesterol levels change over time, and developed a formula for predicting what cholesterol level a person with a given reading at a given age would have years later—assuming that he or she makes no changes in lifestyle. The data can be used to predict the serum cholesterol levels of adults age 20 to 57, the study found.

For example, a 30-year-old woman with a cholesterol level of 155 can expect a level of 188 by age 50 and the borderline high level of 200 at age 56 if no exercise or diet improvements are made.

Researchers found that a man's cholesterol count increases by about two points a year from ages 20 to 30 and one point a year from age 30 to 60, or an increase of 50 points over the 40 years, the report said. A woman's cholesterol level, on the other hand, normally increases by about one and a half points a year from age 20 to 40 and two points a year from age 40 to 60 or 70 points over the 40-year span.

- A University of Chicago study found that young men who smoke or have high cholesterol levels are more likely than others to show signs of heart disease before they reach age 35. One of the study's directors, Dr. Henry McGill, said the study was based on autopsies of about 300 15- to 34-year-old white men who died violent deaths or in accidents. By age 34, one-fourth of the subjects already had what doctors call "raised lesions" in their arteries, representing the beginning of hardening of the arteries.

What does all of this say about Moore's claim of a cholesterol "myth"? Briefly, it says he was wrong.

First, though there is still much that science does not understand about cholesterol, the weight of evidence showing a link between high cholesterol levels and heart disease—both fatal and non-fatal—is too overwhelming to ignore. As a general rule, the higher the cholesterol level, the more a person is at risk.

To the degree that Moore pointed to the need for more research on groups outside the highest-risk group, middle-aged men, that research was already in the pipeline; the heart establishment didn't need Moore to tell it what to do. I don't think researchers can be faulted for focusing most of their research first on the highest-risk group.

There are two basic flaws in Moore's approach to cholesterol, and they're related. The first is that he takes a macroscopic approach, looking at statistics and grand trends—and not at people. Though policy is made with grand trends in mind, it is also based on people—living, breathing individuals with different histories and risk factors, who have to make their own decisions about their cholesterol levels.

Cholesterol is not static; it changes as we age and alter our lifestyle. If I have a cholesterol level of 256 at 42, unless I do something to lower it, I can bet it's going to be higher at 52 and 62 and 72. That means my risk increases with age. If a woman my age has a cholesterol level of 256, by the time she goes through menopause, her cholesterol level will probably be higher than mine and her risk will increase dramatically. And if a teenaged boy has a cholesterol level that's high for his age, he can expect a steadily increasing level throughout his life if he doesn't take steps to lower it.

The second flaw in Moore's approach is that he ignores the differences between patients. I can afford to take some time to try other means than drugs to lower my cholesterol level because I know I have no blockages in my healthy artery. If I had any kind of blockage, I wouldn't delay for a minute. My cholesterol is higher now that I'm eating more healthful foods than it was when I wasn't. There are obviously things going on in my body that are not easy to control. (To be fair, there are people who weigh 150 pounds and have cholesterol levels of 300.) For example, doctors know that if you carry your weight above the waist (an apple), your cholesterol level is higher than if you carry it below your waist (a pear). I'm an apple. That explains why I may get my fanny pinched every once in a great while, but it also helps explain the jump in my cholesterol level.

Similarly, Moore focuses too much on overall cholesterol levels and doesn't pay enough attention to LDL and HDL levels. A Johns Hopkins University study led by Dr. Michael Miller found that too low an HDL level may be at least as bad as a high LDL level. The study of 1,000 patients found 185 men and 47 women who had coronary artery disease even though their total cholesterol was below 200. After excluding patients with recent heart attacks, this left 138 men and 37 women.

The study found that 68 percent of the men and 32 percent of the women had HDL levels below 35. The ongoing Framingham, Massachusetts, heart study found that risk of heart attack rises as HDL level declines; someone with an HDL level of 35 has a 50 percent higher risk than someone with an HDL level of 45.

Moore also ignored the way the heart establishment factors risks other than high cholesterol into its recommendations. Obviously, the more risk factors you have, the more important it is to reduce all of them.

All of this leads to some basic conclusions:

- If your cholesterol is high, lower it.
- If you're still eating a lot of eggs, red meat, ice cream, cream, whole milk, and butter, you should be able to get a noticeable lowering by switching to skim milk and low-fat margarine and cutting back sharply on the eggs and meat.
- Adding foods like oat bran, corn bran, rice bran, beans, and rice could help as well.
- Exercise will raise your HDLs, and there's evidence that monounsaturated fats like olive oil will lower your overall cholesterol without lowering your HDLs.
- If all of that, plus losing weight and generally sticking to the American Heart Association recommended cholesterol and fat levels, doesn't work, or doesn't work enough, it's time for some chemical help.

9

LESSONS

I'm writing this last chapter just a few months before the fifth anniversary of my heart attack. A great deal has changed in that time. Jayne is back in school, Matt's in the Navy, and Dan is practically a teenager. We have a new dog, Tony, a yellow Labrador retriever. I'm writing full time, with about a dozen regular and semi-regular clients, and though it has its ups and downs, I feel more like myself than I have in years. My stress level is coming down, I've lost eight pounds (17 to go), and I started taking lovastatin (Mevacor) to lower my cholesterol. After one month, my cholesterol fell from 241 to 190, and my "bad cholesterol" from 169 to 91. I know I'll be fighting both weight and cholesterol for the rest of my life, but I feel that I'm about to win a round. I've decided the only way I'm going to get all the exercise I need is to be able to do it at home, and I've ordered our own treadmill, which will arrive any day.

I want to end with some advice to readers who either find themselves where I was, or who want to make sure that they don't. I'm not a doctor; I make no claims to give "medical" advice. Consider this a patient's advice, the sort of thing I'd tell a friend.

• First of all, what happened to me can happen to you. We baby boomers may have more of a sense of our own importance, maybe even our own immortality, than other Americans, but we're moving into our peak cardiac years. The lives we've led—fueled by job pressures, junk food, couch-potato status, and stress—make us prime candidates.

• I say this from personal experience, as a son and as a father: if there is a history of heart disease in your family, take it very seriously—it can happen to you. It doesn't have to if you take care of yourself, but you're never too young to start. It amazes me that I know men who are in their late 30s, 40s, or early 50s and are approaching or have passed the age at which their fathers died of a heart attack, yet they have high cholesterol or they smoke and they've never had a stress test. As far as I'm concerned, family history is the first risk factor to consider. If you have other risk factors as well, you're playing with fire. When insurance companies take applications for life insurance, they ask if your parents or any of your brothers and sisters died of a heart attack or cancer before age 60. There must be a reason that they ask that, so if the answer is "Yes," go get a good cardiac checkup. If someone in your family had a heart attack under 50, run, do not walk, to the nearest cardiologist.

• I know this sounds macabre, but make sure you have plenty of life insurance. Buy life insurance on your mortgage. Buy a lot when you're young and it's cheap. Consumer groups tell you not to buy expensive add-on life insurance when you buy a car or take out a loan or open a credit card because it's much cheaper to put the same money in a term insurance policy. It is, but nobody ever does it. When you buy a car, take out life insurance. When you open a credit card, take out life insurance. When you buy a washer and dryer on the installment plan, take out life insurance. It's only money, and it buys peace of mind.

• Know your cholesterol level, and that includes a lipid profile that tells you your LDL and HDL levels. The ratio of total cholesterol to HDL is important; it should be 4.5 to 1, and if it's higher than that, you could have a problem, even if your total cholesterol is below 200. If your total cholesterol is 195, and your HDLs are only 30, that's a 6.5 to 1 ratio and you need to do something about it.*

• Throughout this book, I've written from a man's perspective and with an audience of men in mind. That's only natural; I was writing about my own experience, and most heart attack victims are men. But that's changing, and women aren't immune. The increase in heart attacks among women has come along with the increased number of women in the work force, and I'm sure that's no coincidence. I certainly don't mean that women who don't work out of the home don't have stressful lives; it may well be that workplace stress, perhaps time pressures, takes a different toll on the system. In any event, women, particularly as they approach menopause, need to be concerned about cardiac health.

• If you're having chest pains you don't understand, get to an emergency room immediately. It's better to be embarrassed about a bad case of heartburn or stress and be alive than to avoid an embarrassing situation and be dead.

Good Cholesterol, Bad Cholesterol by Eli Roth and Sandra Streicher (Prima, 1989) is a good reference on the subject.

• If you have chest pains and a doctor tells you your electrocardiogram is fine, don't accept that. An EKG can tell whether you *have had* a heart attack or *are having* one; it can't tell whether you're *about to have* one. You could have a perfect EKG and drop dead on the way out the office door. A treadmill stress test is the best way to tell whether there is a dangerous blockage in your arteries. When the runner Jim Fixx died of a heart attack in his mid-50s, there was a strange debate over whether his running had helped him live five years longer than his father, who had also died of a heart attack, or if his conditioning had killed him because it masked his blockages. As near as I can tell, if he had listened to his doctor and gone for a stress test, it would have shown the blockages, he'd have had a bypass or angioplasty, and he'd probably still be running.

• Don't believe everything you read in the papers or see on TV. As a journalist, I know that's good advice anyway, but it's particularly good advice when it comes to reports on heart research. Headlines don't catch all the details and nuances. For example, I do a lot of work with public opinion figures, and I know that the size and makeup of the sample is important. If one study of 4,000 people says olive oil lowers cholesterol and another study of 36 people says it doesn't, I'm going to be a lot more impressed with the larger study; the smaller sample is almost meaningless. One study got lots of headlines for saying that oat bran does not, in fact, lower cholesterol. The study was conducted on 20 hospital dietitians with an average cholesterol of 186—not exactly typical of either those most at risk for heart attacks or the general population.

• Don't expect a miracle food. Even eating tons of oat bran or drowning all your food in olive oil isn't going to offset the rest of your diet if you don't eat right. *Esquire* columnist Stanley Bing wrote one of the funniest things I've ever read in my life, a piece on the "oat bran puck." He described a day of eating the fattiest, most cholesterol-laden foods imaginable (he described bellying up to the Marriott Cholesterol Bar) and washing them away with an oat bran puck filled with every fiber-rich food known to humanity ("mung to taste") and pots of hot coffee. His point was well taken; there is no magic puck.

• Read the fine print on food labels very carefully. "95% fat free" means 5 percent fat, and that's a lot. Something that blares "No Cholesterol" may be loaded with saturated fat. I've seen frozen Salisbury steak dinners with only 300 calories but with 34 grams of fat—as much as in a lean, one-pound steak.

• Moderation is a wonderful thing. Try to follow too strict a diet, and you'll be miserable and ignore it; follow a moderate diet that allows you a steak once in a while, and you'll stick to it. Drink too much and you'll raise your risk of a heart attack; take a drink now and again and you may relax and help raise your HDLs. Exercise as if you're training for the Olympics and you'll probably end up hurting yourself; follow a nice, steady, moderate exercise program, and you'll live longer.

• The heart, for all the complicated, essential things it does, is a muscle, and it responds like a muscle. If you never take it out for a walk, it will turn into a couch potato, your pulse rate and blood pressure will go up, and so will your risk of heart disease. Give your heart a good workout, get it into and keep it in shape, and it will hum—and it will last you a lot longer.

• Listen to your body; it's sending you messages all day long, and you ignore them at your peril. If you're tired, rest. If you're tense, relax. Do something for fun.

• A positive attitude and a sense of humor are essential. They may not constitute a miracle cure, but they reduce stress, help keep things in perspective, and keep you going.

• It's much easier to picture the world getting along without you while you go on vacation for a week or two when you've seen, "up close and personal," what the world would look like without you for good.

• You can do more damage to yourself than anyone without a lethal weapon can do to you. You can't eliminate stress or anger from your life, but you can regulate them.

• Time is relative. It can be as long or as short as you want. If you start out by putting pressure on yourself about the amount of work you have to do in a certain period of time, you tighten up and you shrink time; because you won't function as efficiently, it takes you longer to do things. If you relax, keep your perspective, and focus on the work rather than the time, time expands; because you're functioning more efficiently, it takes less time to do things. Success breeds success; if you have a number of tasks, the more you finish, no matter how small, the more sense of completion you'll have, the more relaxed you'll become, and the more you'll get done in the same time.

• There's always a choice; whenever you're stressed, frazzled, angry, frustrated, or whatever, you can choose to feel differently. Of course, when you're feeling any of those things, you're least likely to remember that, but it is possible. In the early '70s I did some writing about suicide, and I volunteered for a while for a telephone crisis center. I remember that experts say people dwell on the idea of suicide when they think they have no other choice; when people can be made to realize that there are other alternatives, they stop thinking about killing themselves. The same is true on a much less life-and-death level; you can always feel differently about what's bothering you. I tend to resist that; I figure that if a person has a problem and is not upset, he or she must be psychotic. But not all problems are as serious as we make them out to be, and real problems are not made any better because we're upset. In fact, the more upset we are, the less likely we are to see alternatives and solutions.

• When you have a heart attack, your whole family is a victim. Your spouse and children will be affected in different ways; they need to heal and recover, too, and it will take them as long as it takes you—maybe even longer.

• There are stages in recovery from a heart attack. The stages I went through may not be the same for everyone, but I'm sure they're fairly typical. First comes shock at what's happened to you. That's followed by exhilaration—"I survived." Then comes apprehension—"What's going to happen to me? How will my life change? How can I handle those changes?" The pressures are the greatest at the time the support is the weakest—when you first go home from the hospital. Any help and support you can get at this stage is worth its weight in gold, and the medical community would be advised to pay more attention to this period. As you approach "normalcy," there's a tension between wanting to put the attack behind you and return to things as you knew them and wanting to avoid old bad habits. That tension never goes away; once you've had a heart attack, it's yours, and it stays with you forever.

• There's another way in which a heart attack stays with you forever—you never feel completely safe again. It's as though your body has been invaded, as though you've been mugged or raped. You can go long periods of time without thinking about it, but it always comes back. If you have a pain in your chest, you'll always wonder whether it's your heart. If you're five minutes late, your spouse thinks you've had another heart attack. The tension gets better, but it never goes away.

• When all is said and done, you have to take the primary responsibility for your own recovery because you're the only one who can. No one else can make you exercise, force pills down your throat, monitor every spoonful that goes into your mouth, change your habits of work and play, and make you stop to enjoy life and the people around you. And that's not a burden; once you've made that recovery, you own it, it's yours, something concrete you can hold onto and take pride in and turn to for encouragement. Recovering from a heart attack is such an accomplishment that it's tempting to put it on your résumé.

• The last piece of advice is both simple and ambivalent. Plainly stated, you can recover from a heart attack, even a severe one, even when you're young and half your life is still ahead of you. When I think about a heart attack today, I think of two things. One is the '60s poster that says, "Death is life's way of telling you to slow down." The other is the cliché that the Chinese symbol for "crisis" means both danger and opportunity. A heart attack signals danger, but it also gives you an opportunity—to slow down, to change. The ambivalence comes from this paradox: at one level, of course I'd rather be walking around with an undamaged heart and three blockage-free arteries. And yet, at the same time, I like myself better today than I did five years ago; I'm more mature,

more relaxed, more aware, more open, and healthier—
all because I had a heart attack.

Do I follow all my own advice? Some days more than
others. But I know in a way that I never imagined five
years ago that to the degree that I do follow this advice,
my life will probably be longer and will definitely be
richer.

Appendix A

Diet

_____

Because the chief goal of diet for cardiac concerns is reducing the level of cholesterol in the blood, medical experts are increasingly concerned about the role of saturated fat in stimulating the body's production of cholesterol. The National Cholesterol Education Project (NCEP) says switching to low-fat diets would lower the average American's cholesterol 10 percent and cut incidence of coronary heart disease 20 percent over the next decade.

The NCEP says the biggest decrease in fat intake should come from cutting back on foods rich in saturated fatty acids, like butter, lard, and fatty meats. Saturated fats currently make up about 13.2 percent of an adult's daily calories, well above the 10 percent level recommended by the experts. The average American now gets 34 to 37 percent of his or her diet from all fats; the NCEP recommends this be reduced to no more than 30 percent.

The average American man eats about 435 milligrams of cholesterol per day and the average women about 304.

The expert panel advises cholesterol be limited to 300 milligrams or less per day.

The NCEP says if most Americans follow these guidelines, the average blood cholesterol level of a typical American would drop at least 10 percent, translating into a 20 percent reduction in the incidence of coronary heart disease over the next five to ten years.

A new study shows that lowering the amount of fat in the diet even by a little can go a long way toward reducing the risk of developing new blockages in the coronary arteries.

Dr. David H. Blankenhorn, director of the Atherosclerosis Research Institute at the University of Southern California School of Medicine in Los Angeles, said, "These were not really austere diets. The idea may be out there that you've really got to eat a restricted diet or lose weight. . . . These guys didn't lose weight."

The two-year study examined 82 middle-aged men who had undergone heart bypass surgery and were counseled to reduce their total fat consumption to 26 percent of total calories. They were given angiograms before and after the two-year period, during which they were quizzed semimonthly about all the food they'd eaten in the previous 24 hours. After two years, 18 of the men had developed new fatty deposits in their coronary arteries, and 64 men had not.

Dietary analysis revealed that men who were free of new fatty deposits, or lesions, had reduced their total fat consumption, while the men who developed new lesions had increased total fat consumption. Consumption of saturated fats had gone down in both groups, but it was reduced more in the group with no new lesions; consumption of polyunsaturated fats in both groups had gone up, but consumption in the group with new lesions had gone up more than twice as much as the other group.

This section summarizes recent research on some key areas of diet.

MONOUNSATURATED FATS

Monounsaturated fats like olive oil lower cholesterol, but they also benefit the heart in other ways—they lower both blood pressure and blood sugar, according to a study conducted in Italy.

The study, directed by Dr. Maurizio Trevisan of the State University of New York School of Medicine in Buffalo, examined 4,903 men and women age 20 to 59 in nine communities. It found that those who consumed the most olive oil had the lowest levels of blood cholesterol, blood pressure, and blood glucose.

The study found that diets high in polyunsaturated fats were associated with lower levels of cholesterol and blood glucose, but not with lower blood pressure. Those who ate butter had higher levels of cholesterol, glucose, and blood pressure.

An earlier study led by Dr. Scott Grundy at the University of Texas Health Science Center found that monounsaturated fats were at least as effective as polyunsaturated fats, like sunflower oil, in lowering cholesterol. But, unlike the polyunsaturated fats, the monounsaturated fats reduced only low-density lipoproteins (LDLs), not high-density lipoproteins (HDLs).

FISH OIL

A study of 2,033 men recovering from heart attacks found that those who ate fatty fish two or three times a week were about one-third less likely to die during a two-year follow-up period than those who did not.

Reporting in the British journal *Lancet,* doctors from South Wales said their study found that recovering heart attack patients who consumed 7 to 14 ounces of oily fish, like mackerel or sardines, each week had a 29 percent lower chance of dying than those on other diets. That difference was caused by a substantially lower number of second, killer heart attacks in the fish diet group, researchers said.

However, the study showed that fish oil does not appear to guard against nonfatal heart attacks—both fish and nonfish groups had about the same rate of recurrence.

The Welsh team, headed by Drs. Michael Burr and Ann Fehily, speculated that the Omega-3 fatty acids in fish oil may reduce heart attack severity by lessening the rapid, uneven heartbeats caused by blood clots within the heart. Previous studies have indicated that fish oil reduces clotting and may also slow plaque buildup in the coronary artery, they noted.

William Harris, a fish oil expert at the University of Kansas Medical Center in Kansas City, said he was "pleasantly surprised" by the new findings. "The 29 percent reduction in total mortality was pretty impressive . . . this is the first time I know of that a nutritional intervention that is fairly easy to comply with has worked" to reduce deaths in former heart attack patients, Harris said. "This is really the first hard evidence fish oil can make a difference," he added.

Currently, there is no consensus in the medical community about the value of fish oil in fighting heart disease, Harris said. Short-term studies have found conflicting results on whether fish oil improves the survival of heart patients who undergo balloon angioplasty to open clogged arteries.

In healthy people, the effectiveness of fish oil has generally been gauged by markers thought to be associated with heart disease, such as cholesterol. In the Welsh study, fish oil did not lower cholesterol levels—and its beneficial effects apparently stem from other mechanisms.

"Things may be happening inside the arteries that you

can't take blood samples and measure," Harris said. "Fish oil may be doing important things quietly 'under the cover' where you can't see them happening."

Unlike past studies that gave patients large doses of fish oil, Harris noted that the fish intake recommended by the Welsh doctors was "fairly tolerable" for most people. About 14 percent of patients in the study opted, with doctor's permission, to substitute fish oil capsules for their required quota of fish.

High doses of fish oil can pose a threat of bleeding and can also cause weight gain. The men in the study, who were all under 70, gained an average of about 1.3 pounds over two years no matter what diet they ate.

The Welsh study did not look at whether fish oil can guard healthy people against killer heart attacks. But Harris observed, "One would be tempted to draw the conclusion that if it protects from a second fatal heart attack, it may protect from a first."

At the very least, Harris said doctors should recommend that recovering heart attack patients eat more fish, "and increasing oily fish intake would be more appropriate." He added, "I also don't think there is a strong argument to keep people from taking a few fish oil supplements if they don't like fish."

COFFEE

Three major studies on coffee and the heart were done in 1989 and 1990:

A Scandinavian study found that filtered coffee, by far the favorite among United States coffee drinkers, may also be the most healthful for the heart. It found a strong link between rising cholesterol levels and boiled coffee, a brewing method popular in Scandinavia.

People who boiled their coffee every day for nine weeks had a ten percent rise in their cholesterol levels, but when they stayed with filtered coffee, their cholesterol levels remained steady.

Dr. Diederick E. Grobbee of Erasmus University Medical School in the Netherlands, said that the latest findings raise concerns that percolators might also have a bad effect on cholesterol. "Without having tested the possibility," he said, "there is some reason to believe it might be somewhat similar."

In the study, 107 young adults with normal cholesterol levels drank filtered coffee for three weeks. Then they were randomly assigned to drink four to six cups a day of boiled coffee, four to six cups of filtered coffee, or no coffee at all. After nine weeks, their total cholesterol levels rose 10 percent after they switched to boiled coffee, but the cholesterol levels were unchanged in those who used filtered coffee or those who abstained.

Grobbee offered three possible explanations for why boiled coffee seems to raise cholesterol:

- It's made with hotter water than drip coffee.
- The water stays in contact with the coffee grounds longer.
- Filters screen out some cholesterol-raising substance in coffee.

A Stanford University study found that decaffeinated coffee tends to raise LDL levels slightly. Dr. H. Robert Superko said researchers studied a group of 181 men who drank their usual three to six cups of coffee a day for two months. At the end of the two months, one group stayed on regular coffee, one switched to decaffeinated coffee, and one stayed away from coffee altogether. At the end of the second two months, those who had quit drinking coffee or stayed with regular coffee had slightly lower LDL levels, while those who had switched to decaffeinated coffee had slightly higher LDL levels, some as much as five percent higher. Superko speculated that the difference may come from the kind of beans used to make the different coffees; the regular coffee was made with arabica beans and the decaffeinated coffee used was made with stronger robusta beans.

A Norwegian study found that cholesterol levels rose the more cups of coffee were drunk daily, and that mortality rose steadily in men drinking more than two cups a day. There were fewer deaths among women.

The study, the largest yet of links between coffee drinking and heart disease, involved 38,564 men and women in Norway. The researchers, from the National Health Screening Service in Oslo, said, "Coffee may affect mortality from coronary heart disease over and above its effect in raising cholesterol concentrations."

Altogether, 168 men and 16 women died of heart disease during the four- to nine-year follow-up period of the study.

The Norwegian researchers studied 19,398 men and 19,166 women ages 35 to 54 from 1977 to 1982. The subjects reported no symptoms of cardiovascular disease or diabetes and later were followed until the end of 1986. During the follow-up period, 168 men and 16 women died of coronary heart disease, the researchers said.

Of the men who died, 130 drank between five and nine cups of coffee a day. There were six deaths among men who drank one or two cups a day and three deaths among men who drank less than one cup, the study found. Among women, the researchers said, an excess risk was found only for those who drank seven or more cups of coffee every day.

ALCOHOL

There is still some conflict among research studies on the relationship of alcohol and heart disease, but this seems to be the case: more than two drinks a day is clearly a problem because that much alcohol can raise blood pressure. It can also lead to cirrhosis of the liver, throat cancer, and other problems, and too much alcohol is clearly associated with accidents. But one or two drinks a day may actually raise HDL and lower LDL levels and reduce stress levels.

EGGS

The American Heart Association says Americans may eat four eggs a week instead of three as part of a healthful diet in light of the United States Department of Agriculture's new estimate of the amount of cholesterol in eggs.

Previously, the USDA said one egg had 274 milligrams of cholesterol, but more accurate readings lowered that level to 213 milligrams.

Dr. John LaRosa, chairman of the AHA nutrition committee, said, "This viewpoint does not represent a change in the AHA's dietary guidelines—the nutrition committee still recommends a maximum of 300 milligrams of dietary cholesterol a day."

LaRosa said the four-egg-a-week recommendation includes "'invisible' yolks consumed in baked goods and other prepared foods."

BRAN

For the past few years, scientists have been urging people to eat oat bran as a means of lowering cholesterol. A study released in early 1990 challenged that view, but other evidence suggests that oat bran does help lower cholesterol —as do other brans and foods.

The new research claimed that people who eat a lot of oat bran have less cholesterol in their blood simply because they eat less saturated fat and cholesterol. Dr. Frank Sacks, a coauthor of the study conducted at Brigham and Women's Hospital in Boston, said people's cholesterol levels dropped just as much when they ate food made with low-fiber white flour and Cream of Wheat as it did with heavy intake of oat bran, because fat consumption went down.

The study was conducted on 20 volunteers, most of them hospital dietitians. Using dietitians as test subjects meant the researchers had a healthy group who already largely followed recommended diets. Their cholesterol levels averaged 186.

Dietitian Linda Van Horn at Northwestern University, who had previously found that substituting oat bran for other carbohydrates in the diet lowered blood cholesterol levels by three percent, said, "With their small sample size and without the dietary control necessary to monitor the situation, I don't know what this means."

Many experts dismiss the new study on the grounds that they understand the mechanism through which oat bran lowers cholesterol—it flushes bile acids from the body, forcing the liver to take cholesterol out of the bloodsteam to replace them.

But if oat bran helps lower cholesterol, it is not alone. New studies have shown that corn bran and rice bran also lower cholesterol, as do barley and dried beans.

THE NIBBLING DIET
AND CHOLESTEROL

People who nibble all day instead of eating three square meals have significantly lower blood cholesterol levels, according to a University of Toronto study. The researchers said this means that cholesterol levels "may be lowered by increasing meal frequency alone, with no alteration in the nature or amount of the food eaten."

However, they said they did not advocate putting people on the diet they tested, which they describe as "an extreme model of nibbling."

In the study, directed by Dr. David J. A. Jenkins, seven men each ate 2,500 calories a day. For one two-week period, they got their food in three ordinary-size meals. But for another two weeks, they got the same amount of calories in 17 snacks eaten one per hour.

The nibbling diet lowered their total cholesterol levels by 9 percent and their LDL levels by 14 percent. The researchers said that what they found "is consistent with the claim that increasing meal frequency while maintaining a constant caloric intake may have a role in the prevention of heart disease."

The researchers speculated that nibbling might somehow help by lowering insulin levels or prompting the liver to make less cholesterol.

APPENDIX B

EXERCISE

———

This is what exercise can do for you:

- It improves your heart's condition and efficiency, lowering your pulse rate.
- It lowers your blood pressure.
- It raises your HDL levels.
- It turns fat into muscle.
- It reduces your appetite and helps your body process food more efficiently.
- It raises your blood volume, which reduces stress on your heart.
- It reduces depression and makes you feel better.

And, now, there's evidence that just a little exercise can lengthen your life. That's the major finding of a 15-year study of more than 13,000 men and women.

"You don't have to be an athlete; you don't have to do hours of vigorous exercise every week to get some obvious benefits," according to Steven N. Blair, an epidemiologist and coauthor of the study published in the *Journal of the American Medical Association.* Blair said those who don't exercise at all can get the greatest benefit from exercise. He said 30 to 45 minutes of brisk walking each day "will produce the moderate levels [of fitness] that are associated with much lower death rates."

The Institute for Aerobics Research in Dallas, which conducted the study, examined 10,224 men and 3,120 women for an average of more than eight years. Of those, 240 men and 43 women died during the study.

Among men who were the least fit, the death rate was 64 per 10,000 person-years, compared with 16.6 among the most fit group. A person-year equals the number of people studied multiplied by the number of years they were followed. Among women, deaths dropped from 39.5 per 10,000 person-years to 8.5 per 10,000 among the most fit.

Heart-disease death rates among men fell from 24.6 per 10,000 person-years among the least fit to 3.1 for those in the two most fit groups. For women, heart-disease death rates dropped from 7.4 to 0.8.

The study also suggested that increased fitness may help compensate for other factors that might shorten life, Blair said. For example, people in the study who had high blood pressure but were otherwise highly fit lived longer than people with low blood pressure who were inactive.

Despite exercise's benefits, only 8 percent of Americans meet recommended exercise goals, according to the U.S. Centers for Disease Control (CDC). In 1980, the Department of Health and Human Services set a goal for 60 percent of the 18-to-65 population to be involved in regular vigorous physical activity by 1990, the CDC said. Despite that, only 10 percent to 20 percent were participating at the level suggested in a progress report in 1985.

Many physicians recommend an exercise regimen of at least three times per week and at least 20 minutes per session. Data from a survey conducted between 1984 and

1987 showed only 8 percent were participating at that level, the CDC said.

The Health Department also set a goal calling for 50 percent of people under 65 to participate in such lower-intensity physical activity as swimming or walking by 1990. In 1975, about 35 percent of adults reported taking regular walks or comparable physical activity, a number that rose to 46 percent in 1985. But only 8 percent of them engaged in the activities "long enough or often enough" to satisfy federal recommendations, the CDC said.

The relationship between good health and exercise is well-documented, the CDC said. "Evidence indicates that regular physical activity reduces the incidence of and/or is otherwise beneficial to many medical conditions—including coronary heart disease, colon cancer, osteoporosis, hypertension, depression, diabetes mellitus, and obesity," the report said.

The CDC said two of the objectives appear to have been met. The Health Department set a 1990 goal for 25 percent of companies with more than 500 workers to offer fitness programs. The CDC said the number of companies offering exercise programs jumped from 3 percent in 1979 to at least 30 percent in 1985. An objective calling for 50 percent of doctors to ask fitness questions in their initial examination of new patients also appears to have been met, the CDC said.

Here are some of the other "Objectives for the Nation" published in 1980:

- Half of Americans 65 and older should walk, swim, or engage in other "appropriate" aerobic exercise at least three times a week. A 1985 survey showed that although 46 percent of older Americans said they walked for exercise, just 8 percent met the three-times-a-week, 20-minute level.

- More than 90 percent of youngsters 10–17 should participate three times a week in 20-minute sessions of vigorous exercise. A 1984 survey found only 66 percent of children exercised at that level.

- More than 60 percent of children 10–17 should participate in daily school physical education programs. A 1984 survey placed the figure at 36 percent, up by only 3 percent from a 1974 survey.
- More than 70 percent of U.S. adults should know that cardiovascular health is best promoted by exercising at least three times a week, for 20 minutes or more, and at a level that makes heart rate and breathing "a lot faster," but not so much that talking is impossible. A 1985 survey found that fewer than 40 percent got those questions right.

A survey conducted for *Prevention* magazine found that middle-aged women with college degrees have the most healthful lifestyles. The survey also found that white, male, blue-collar workers have the worst health habits.

The report, "The Fit and the Fat," found a sizable group of people who want to be healthy but lack the resources, both personal and financial. Many others know what to do to be healthy but lack motivation, said Thomas Dybdahl, study director. The study, based on a survey of 1,250 randomly selected Americans, was conducted by Louis Harris Associates.

The survey categorized Americans into the following groups:

The *"young and reckless"* (68 million). They know what healthful practices are but make little effort to follow them. They pay little heed to nutrition, especially fat consumption, are only average at getting medical care, and have a poor record for using auto seat belts. They do however, exercise regularly. A majority are men. They are younger than the national average and have slightly higher than average education and income levels.

The *"healthy and wealthy"* (45 million). They are careful with their diets, limit fat, and make sure they get enough fiber, vitamins, and minerals. They get regular medical tests, maintain proper weight, wear seat belts, and exercise. More than half in this group are women, and they are largely in middle age. Members of this group are likely to have college degrees, high incomes, and professional or managerial jobs.

The *"sedentary but striving"* (14.5 million). They are overweight but want to do better. They have good records for avoiding salt, fat, and cholesterol but still have serious weight problems, with 77 percent of the group overweight. They know it, and about half are trying to lose weight. However, they exercise little. This group does get medical checkups, drinks little, and has good records for home and auto safety. Nearly two-thirds are women. They are older than the national average, are more likely to be minorities, and have the lowest income levels.

The *"safe and satisfied"* (13 million). They tend to have a healthful lifestyle but show little inclination to do better. They limit the fat, salt, and sugar in their diets but are below average in watching cholesterol. This group has the best record for exercising and does well at maintaining the proper weight. However, they are below average for dental visits, sleep less than other groups, and have high stress levels. They are divided almost evenly between men and women. The largest share is over 50, they are slightly below average in education and income, and many hold unskilled jobs.

The *"fat and frustrated"* (13 million). They want to be healthy but don't know what to do. This group has the largest number of members trying to lose weight, and the fewest who succeed. In nutritional habits they are about average, yet 88 percent are overweight. Their rate for exercising is less than half the national average. They have high stress levels. They are mostly women, slightly older than average, more likely to be minorities, and have the lowest education level of any group.

The *"confused and indifferent"* (9 million). They have limited knowledge of what constitutes a healthful life-style and don't care. They have the worst dietary habits, eating lots of fat, salt, and sugar. They rarely have medical checks, and 74 percent are overweight. This group has more nondrinkers than the national average and a poor record for seat belt use. The majority are men, largely whites, with lower than average education and income levels; many hold blue-collar jobs.

Appendix C

Medical Updates

——

Heart disease remains the number-one killer in America. But death rates from heart disease have decreased dramatically over the past three decades and are likely to decrease further throughout the 1990s.

No one can point with certainty to any one factor that is responsible for the decreasing heart disease death rate. It's likely that a combination of factors—more awareness, better diet and exercise, less smoking, new drugs and surgical techniques—are responsible.

A national health study released in 1989 said heart disease accounted for 36 percent of all deaths in the nation during 1986. The survey, conducted by the national Centers for Disease Control, said there were 765,490 deaths from heart disease that year.

"There is one less coronary [heart attack] every minute in this country," according to Dr. Claude Lenfant, director of the National Heart, Lung, and Blood Institute. He said the decline in heart attacks in the United States started in the 1960s, when the rate of death from cardiac disease was more than 400 per 100,000 persons. The rate is dropping at a steady annual rate and now is about 330 per 100,000 persons. "It keeps going down and there is no sign of its leveling off," Lenfant says.

Despite this decline, however, "the U.S. still has one of the highest rates in the world," according to Dr. William T. Friedewald, associate director for disease prevention at the National Institutes of Health.

To put the decline in the U.S. death rate for heart disease in more human terms, if the death rate in 1989 were the same as in 1963, 420,000 more people would have died.

One of the negative sides of the trend is that heart disease is increasingly becoming a blue-collar disease. Better educated Americans have done more to change to a more healthful lifestyle; in particular, blue-collar workers are more likely to smoke, although their smoking rate is decreasing.

What follows is a collection of summaries of reports of medical studies related to heart disease that were published during 1989 and early 1990. They show both the pace with which new information becomes available and the conflicts that sometimes emerge.

ANGIOPLASTY

The routine use of balloon angioplasty following a heart attack and the use of clot-dissolving drugs do not improve chances of survival and may often be unnecessary, according to a major study of more than 3,000 patients at 14 medical centers.

The study compared the treatment of 1,636 heart attack patients who received angioplasty and 1,626 who were treated with drugs. It found that 9.7 percent of the patients treated only with drugs and 10.9 percent of those treated with angioplasty had a second heart attack or died.

The use of clot-dissolving drugs—such as tissue plasminogen activator (TPA) or streptokinase—has dramatically improved survival rates of heart attack victims. The drugs dissolve the blood clots that form during a heart attack and reopen blocked arteries, although 20 to 30 percent of arteries will either never open or will become blocked again.

Many hospitals have routinely followed up use of clot-dissolving drugs with angioplasty if an angiogram shows the artery is blocked. In 1988, 84,000 angioplasties were performed. Angioplasty has its risks; about five percent of the time, it will damage the artery and necessitate an emergency bypass. In 20 to 30 percent of the cases, the area will become blocked again and the procedure will have to repeated.

Angioplasty is effective in treating angina. In the study, 13 percent of those treated only with drugs later needed angioplasty to relieve angina symptoms.

The study director was Dr. Eugene Braunwald, chairman of medicine at Harvard Medical School's Brigham and Women's Hospital and Beth Israel Hospital.

BYPASS SURGERY

Odds of surviving a coronary bypass operation increased greatly between 1969 and 1984 because of improved surgical techniques.

"Patients who benefited most were those with more severe coronary disease, those who had the worst prognosis, or those who were operated on more recently," said Dr. Robert Califf of Duke University Medical Center in Durham, North Carolina.

"The latter association is probably the result of improvements in surgical and medical procedures in recent years, improvements which . . . are probably characteristic of most medical centers in the United States," Califf continued.

The study found one-year surgical survival rates improved from 84 percent in 1970 to 95 percent in 1984 and five-year rates went from 76 percent in 1970 to 89 percent in 1980.

The study examined 5,809 patients—including 2,962 who underwent bypass operations to replace narrowed arteries. It indicated that surgical survival improved progressively and was significantly better for most heart patients than other forms of medical therapy—regardless of such factors as age and heart muscle pain.

Another new study says coronary bypass surgery can help victims of heart disease live better and longer even after they reach their 80s and that no one should be denied the operation simply because of age. However, doctors cautioned that this common form of surgery should be limited to folks who are healthy and independent except for serious chest pain.

"All 80-year-olds are not created equal," said Dr. Gail E. Darling. "People with a lot of other illnesses are not considered good candidates for bypass." But if the patient is otherwise in good shape, she said, "age alone should not be a factor in the decision to proceed with coronary bypass surgery."

Darling, a heart surgeon, based her recommendation on a review of 159 octogenarians who underwent bypass surgery in the past 12 years at the Mayo Clinic. Before the operations, 97 percent of the patients had severe, disabling chest pain that occurred while they were resting or performing such simple activities as cooking or walking. Afterward, most felt dramatic relief from their symptoms and could lead more active lives.

An estimated 284,000 bypass operations were performed in the United States in 1986. Darling said that even though the surgery has become relatively common for people in their 70s, many doctors are still reluctant to perform it on older folks.

The main drawback to the surgery for people in their 80s was a relatively high death rate of 11 percent. However, if the patients survived long enough to be discharged from the hospital, they did relatively well. Overall, 84 percent of those undergoing surgery survived at least one year, and 70 percent were still alive after five years. Darling said this was as good as typical survival for people that age and better than what would be expected for those with serious heart disease.

Between 1977 and 1983, less than one-half of one percent of all bypass patients at the Mayo Clinic were over 80. Since then, this has grown to about three percent.

ASPIRIN

Doctors have known for a number of years that aspirin helps prevent second heart attacks; now they have findings that it also cuts the risk of a first heart attack in men over 50.

The Physicians' Health Study, directed by Dr. Charles H. Hennekens of Brigham and Women's Hospital in Boston, found that men who took a single aspirin every other day had a 44 percent reduction in their risk of heart attacks. However, the benefits were limited to those over age 50, who cut their risk about in half.

"We have a clear-cut, conclusive benefit on reducing a first heart attack," said Hennekens. He said people should not start taking regular aspirin unless they consult first with a doctor or other health professional. In helping make a decision, doctors should consider a patient's other risk factors, such as blood pressure, cholesterol level, and family history of heart disease.

In an editorial accompanying the report in *The New England Journal of Medicine,* Dr. Valentin Fuster and others from Mount Sinai Medical Center in New York wrote that "aspirin appears to be beneficial in the prevention of a first myocardial infarction [heart attack], at least in men over the age of 50, and it has its largest effect in those with uncontrolled risk factors."

Aspirin works by making the blood less likely to clot. Heart attacks usually occur when clots form in the coronary arteries, choking off the heart's blood supply.

The study was conducted on 22,071 men doctors. They were given packs of pills and randomly assigned to take aspirin, beta carotene, or placebos.

Here are some of the findings:

- Aspirin users were slightly more likely to have strokes, but the number was too small to be statistically meaningful.

- There was no overall decrease in cardiovascular deaths among those taking aspirin, but the study would have had to continue to the year 2000 or beyond to show any impact on mortality.

- The benefits of aspirin appeared to be greatest among those with low cholesterol levels.

BLOOD PRESSURE

Patients with high blood pressure who drop their pressure too rapidly face a higher risk of heart attacks, according to a study conducted by the Albert Einstein Medical College of Yeshiva University.

The study, released in August 1989, examined 1,765 members of the Building Service 32B-J welfare fund between 1973 and 1987. It described a decrease of less than 7 milliliters of mercury as small, a decrease of 7 to 17 milliliters as moderate, and a decrease over 17 milliliters as large. It found that 0.9 percent of the group with a moderate decline, 3.1 percent of the group with a large drop, and 3.7 percent of the group with a small drop had heart attacks during the period of the study.

The head of the research team, Dr. Michael Alderman, speculated that a large drop in blood pressure might reduce the flow of blood to the heart in people with hardening of the arteries, depriving the heart of oxygen.

Doctors classify high blood pressure as mild if the diastolic (bottom) number is 90 to 104, moderate if it is 105 to 115, and severe if it is above 115. Alderman says he believes that the optimal reduction is 10 to 12 points for those with mild hypertension and up to 17 for those with moderate hypertension. But he said more studies are needed to determine the optimal reduction. Dr. Claude Lenfant, director of the National Heart, Lung, and Blood Institute, has called for such studies.

ANXIETY

Thousands of people with perfectly healthy hearts are living as virtual "cardiac cripples" because of chest pains caused by untreated anxiety or panic disorders. At the same time, thousands of other people, mostly women, are being treated for psychiatric problems when they are actually suffering from an unusual form of heart disease.

Francis Kane, Jr., professor of psychiatry at the Baylor College of Medicine in Houston, says people in the first group avoid exertion and fear they might have heart disease even after medical tests show their hearts are normal.

Kane and his colleagues surveyed 371 people who had complained of chest pain or other apparent heart trouble, but who showed no sign of disease when tested with a procedure called an angiogram. Despite the angiogram findings, 56 percent of the people were unsure about whether they had heart disease, 45 percent feared that exertion would be dangerous, and 32 percent said their physical activities were limited.

Sixty-nine percent of the people qualified for diagnosis of panic attacks or another anxiety disorder, based on their answers to the survey, said Kane. He reported his findings at a meeting of the American Psychiatric Association.

More than one million Americans have panic attacks, which inflict sudden bouts of intense terror for no apparent reason, according to the American Psychiatric Association. About half had been told their symptoms were due to stress, but only 4 percent were told to seek mental health treatment and only 17 percent were given tranquilizers, Kane said.

Kane said about 540,000 angiograms were performed in 1984, and the annual total has probably risen since; about 10 percent to 45 percent of such tests find no sign of heart disease.

Symptoms of chest pain, palpitation, breathlessness, and fear of fainting tended to be reported by people who also appeared to suffer from panic attacks, the survey showed.

The survey also found that generalized anxiety disorder was linked to persistent chest pain and belief that one had suffered a heart attack. Fifty-five percent of the sample believed they had suffered a heart attack, although only 2 percent had been told that in the past. Generalized anxiety disorder is characterized by unrealistic or excessive anxiety and worry about two or more circumstances of one's life for six months or more.

The second misdiagnosed group consists of tens of thousands of American women who are being misdiagnosed as suffering from psychiatric disorders when they are in fact suffering from an unusual form of heart disease. The women, who have chest pain but no signs of heart disease by conventional tests, are suffering from a treatable disorder of the small arteries, according to Dr. Richard Cannon of the National Heart, Lung, and Blood Institute in Bethesda, Maryland. "Many have been mislabeled as neurotic or hysterical women," Cannon said. "They truly have a pain syndrome."

Cannon said the disorder afflicts up to 100,000 Americans each year, most of them women. Among their symptoms is a condition Cannon calls "sensitive heart," in which they experience sharp pain when test probes are threaded into arteries near their hearts. Such probes usually are painless, he said.

Cannon's studies show that many of the patients are suffering from a disorder he calls microvascular angina, in which blood flow may be blocked in very tiny arteries that nourish the heart. The arteries are too small to show up on angiograms, he said. The condition has sometimes been called "syndrome X," because its cause is unknown. It may be common in men, but it occurs in middle age and later, when many men have already developed coronary artery blockages. Those blockages hide underlying microvascular angina, Cannon said.

A variety of treatments, including many standard heart drugs, is used to relieve the pain, according to Cannon.

The patients are identified in part because they have reduced flow of blood to the heart, Cannon said. Studies have shown that the patients appear to have a disorder of the so-called "smooth muscle" in arteries. The smooth muscle causes arteries to tighten and relax as they help regulate blood pressure and blood flow.

The patients are unusually sensitive to drugs that constrict the blood vessels, and somewhat insensitive to drugs that relax blood vessels, Cannon went on. They also commonly have disorders of the esophagus and an asthma-like condition in the bronchial tubes. The esophagus and the bronchial tubes contain smooth muscle. The disorder could be caused by some defect in the smooth muscle itself, or it could be a problem in the portions of the brain and nervous system that regulate the contraction and relaxation of smooth muscle, Cannon continued.

Although microvascular angina is not a psychiatric condition, some psychiatric drugs appear to relieve the chest pain, perhaps because they alleviate a disorder in the nervous system's regulation of the smooth muscle, Cannon said.

CARBON MONOXIDE

Levels of carbon monoxide considered safe by federal air quality standards can trigger a potentially dangerous oxygen shortage in the hearts of people with coronary artery disease, according to a study conducted by the St. Louis University School of Medicine. The study found effects at carbon monoxide levels equal to those in a room full of cigarette smokers.

The study found a decrease in the amount of work that people with heart disease could perform when their carboxyhemoglobin levels—the combination of carbon monoxide and hemoglobin—reached 2 percent. Hemoglobin ordinarily combines with oxygen and carries it throughout the body. But carbon monoxide binds with hemoglobin even more tightly than oxygen does. So when people breathe carbon monoxide, it cuts down the amount of oxygen in their blood, and high doses are fatal.

In general, standards set by the U.S. Environmental Protection Agency allow enough carbon monoxide in the air to take up 2 percent of the blood's hemoglobin. "What we have shown with this paper is that it's beyond any doubt that there is a documented effect at 2 percent, which frankly was a surprise to us," said Dr. Thomas E. Dahms. "It's such a small amount that one would not think you could see that kind of change."

Federal health surveys have found that 5 percent to 10 percent of all nonsmoking Americans have this much carboxyhemoglobin in their blood at any time. The two chief sources of carbon monoxide in the air are cigarette smoke and engine fumes.

Dahms said a nonsmoker in a closed room with 20 smokers would breathe enough carbon monoxide to have about a 2 percent carboxyhemoglobin level. Someone who smokes a pack of cigarettes a day has levels between 4 percent and 8 percent.

The study was performed on 63 men with coronary artery disease. They exercised on a treadmill while breathing ordinary air or air that increased their carboxyhemoglobin levels to 2 percent or 4 percent. At 2 percent carbon monoxide levels, they could do 5 percent less exercise before their hearts showed signs of oxygen deprivation, and at 4 percent levels, they could do 12 percent less exercise. They also developed chest pain sooner with increasing levels of carbon monoxide.

As people exercise, their hearts demand more oxygen. In people with healthy hearts, their arteries can expand to deliver more oxygen-rich blood, and small amounts of carbon monoxide have little effect. But when people have heart disease, clogged arteries don't expand properly. Carbon monoxide can make an important difference by lowering the oxygen load of the blood that gets through.

DOCTOR TALK

Doctors dehumanize their patients when discussing medical treatment by unconsciously using a language that differs greatly from ordinary speech, a researcher says.

During her 19-month study, University of Michigan sociologist Renee Anspach observed doctors in two intensive-care nurseries and in an obstetrics and gynecology ward. She also analyzed written records, such as discharge summaries and operation reports.

She said that while the speech patterns are unintentional, they remove human judgment from medical decisions, distancing doctors from the consequences of their actions. "The language protects those who use it from public scrutiny and supports the profession's natural impulse to protect itself in a climate of increasing malpractice suits," she said.

She cited an example involving the treatment of a woman with cervical cancer. The doctor said, "No pap smear was performed at the time of the initial visit."

"In that case, not performing the pap smear was a serious error in medical management. But by using the passive voice, the presenter softened the accusation by drawing attention toward the error and away from the person responsible," Anspach said.

Anspach said the language conventions reinforce the world view of a doctor. "It's almost a cliché . . . but the real actors in the drama are not human beings but their organ systems and diseases."

ARTERY REPAIR

Researchers have produced genetically engineered cells that grow inside blood vessels and might one day be able to repair the damaged arteries that lead to heart attacks. The cells, used so far only in animals, take root in arteries and form a new inner lining, said Dr. Elizabeth Nabel of the University of Michigan.

"This is the beginning of a new approach to treatment of cardiovascular disease," Nabel told the American Heart Association's annual science writers' forum.

Such cells might be made to flower inside the arteries and dispense a regular supply of insulin for diabetics, or blood-clotting factors for hemophiliacs, she said. Experiments in the animals have established the feasibility of the approach, although numerous problems must be solved before such cells could be used in humans, she continued.

Habel and her colleagues have so far shown that endothelial cells, which line the arteries, can be genetically altered to incorporate genes related to heart disease or other ailments. They have also shown that such cells, when implanted in a pig's artery, will survive and grow.

The genetically altered endothelial cells have the important advantage that they can be induced to grow in a specific place in the arteries where, for example, hardening of the arteries, or atherosclerosis, is occurring.

SUBSTANCE REDUCES CLOT DESTRUCTION

A cholesterol-carrying particle in the blood may encourage heart attacks by hampering the body's ability to destroy blood clots, according to reports by two teams of researchers working independently.

They found that in the test tube, the particle known as lipoprotein (a) interfered with a key step in clot destruction. Clots trigger heart attacks by plugging narrowed arteries, and one researcher said they may encourage the narrowing of the arteries in the first place. The studies appeared in the British journal *Nature*.

Lipoprotein (a) resembles LDL. It is also associated with atherosclerosis and heart attacks, scientists from the Research Institute of Scripps Clinic in La Jolla, California, and the University of Chicago noted in their *Nature* report.

They followed up on the earlier discovery that one component of the lipoprotein (a) particle strongly resembles a blood protein called plasminogen. Plasminogen plays a key role in the destruction of blood clots, once it binds to other proteins called receptors. The receptors appear on blood cells and the lining of blood vessels.

Researchers found that in the test tube, lipoprotein (a) also bound to those receptors, interfering with the plasminogen binding. So in the body, that interference may hamper the destruction of clots, they suggested.

Scientists from Cornell University Medical College and Rockefeller University in New York reported the same results. They also found evidence of lipoprotein (a) accumulations in the atherosclerotic buildup in blood vessels.

Katherine Hajjar, study coauthor from Cornell, said some scientists suspect that repeated clot formation may predispose a blood vessel to atherosclerosis. So high levels of lipoprotein (a) may encourage atherosclerosis by hampering a vessel's ability to fight clot formation, she said.

The test-tube results make it logical to suspect that lipoprotein (a) may hamper clot destruction in humans, said John Albers of the University of Washington School of Medicine.

For more evidence, scientists should follow people with different levels of lipoprotein (a) to see if they show different rates of clot-induced heart attacks and strokes, Albers said.

WOMEN AND HEART ATTACK RECOVERY

Contrary to previous findings, women survive as well as men after heart attacks if age and illnesses are taken into account.

"Merely being a woman in and of itself does not appear

to be a risk factor" in connection with heart attacks, said lead researcher Dr. Nicholas H. Fiebach of Yale University School of Medicine.

Fiebach and his colleagues explored the issue after two previous studies yielded conflicting results. The new study involved 332 women and 790 men who had suffered heart attacks, and it found that 29 percent of the women and 23 percent of the men died within the three years after the attack.

But "when we did a statistical analysis that took into account differences in age, diabetes, and hypertension, the differences in mortality weren't there anymore," Fiebach said.

Heart disease is the leading killer of men and women, but women tend to be stricken when they are older and have more health problems, Fiebach continued.

Women were more critically ill when they were admitted to the hospital, and a greater proportion of them died there than did men, the researchers found. After being discharged from the hospital, however, the women's adjusted death rate appeared to be a little better than men's, though the difference was not statistically significant, Fiebach said. That finding is consistent with the fact that women in general tend to outlive men, he said.

SHOVELING SNOW AND GETTING OUT OF BED

Climbing out of bed in the middle of the night can be "a risky moment" for the heart, but shoveling snow may not be as dangerous as people have long believed, according to two new studies.

In one, researchers monitored the hearts of people with coronary artery disease while they slept. If they had to get out of bed in the night, their hearts often experienced potentially harmful periods of ischemia—a temporary shortage of blood.

"It seems that jumping out of bed and running around to do something is a risky moment that we should think about," said Dr. Andrew P. Selwyn of Brigham and Women's Hospital in Boston.

On the other hand, researchers at the Medical College of Wisconsin found that for active, physically fit people with heart disease, shoveling snow is probably no riskier than other moderate exercise.

"The feeling over the years has been that we should baby these people," said Sara M. Dougherty, an exercise physiologist who conducted the study. "We want to get away from that. Shoveling is not for everyone. But to say no one can shovel is just as much an error." However, she cautioned that people with heart trouble should not shovel unless they have taken a treadmill test and consulted their doctor.

In the Boston study, directed by Joan Barry, 30 people with heart disease wore heart monitors while they slept. Twenty-one of them got up at night, usually to go to the bathroom, a total of 36 times. On 24 of these occasions, their hearts showed signs of painless ischemia.

Selwyn theorizes that the blood vessels may be slow to adapt to the heart's changing demands when people stand up after lying down. Earlier studies have shown similar ischemic episodes when people climb out of bed in the morning. Selwyn said it may be possible, with drugs such as beta blockers that fight ischemia, to control these activities' effects on the heart.

TRANSCENDENTAL MEDITATION AND LONGEVITY

Elderly people who learned Transcendental Meditation (TM) were more likely than those using two other meditative techniques to still be living after three years. TM was also more effective in lowering blood pressure and improving on several measures of mental functioning.

The Harvard University study was presented in the

Journal of Personality and Social Psychology published by the American Psychological Association.

The study included 73 volunteers, with an average age of 81, from eight homes for the elderly. They were assigned randomly to learn TM, another technique called mindfulness training, a simple relaxation program, or no training at all. Each technique was practiced during the 12-week experiment for 20 minutes twice daily with the eyes closed.

Three years later, the 20 taught TM were still alive. Survival rates in the other groups were 88 percent, 65 percent, and 77 percent, respectively.

TM induces "a distinctively deep state of rest" while the mind is alert but "in a very settled, quiet state," said coauthor Charles Alexander, now an associate professor of psychology at Maharishi International University in Fairfield, Iowa. Students there practice TM as part of the curriculum, Alexander said.

The "mindfulness training" in the study was not the Buddhist technique of the same name. Instead, it was designed to stimulate creation of ideas or new perspectives through a verbal exercise and a challenge to think about topics in new and creative ways.

Alexander attributed the findings to TM's combination of high wakefulness, which he said combats atrophy of the mind and the body, and deep restfulness, which he said releases stress from the nervous system and leads to reduced "wear and tear" on mind and body. He said the study suggests TM should be combined with standard Western medicine, not replace it.

BODY FAT DISTRIBUTION AFFECTS CHOLESTEROL LEVEL

It's healthier to be shaped like a pear than an apple, and now experts believe they know why: Cholesterol levels are closely linked with where people carry their fat.

Researchers have long noticed that folks with fat posteriors tend to have healthier hearts than those with big guts, but the reason for this was unclear.

A new study offers a possible explanation. It shows that people with beefy hips and trim waists have higher levels of a protective form of cholesterol called HDL than do those with potbellies and small behinds.

"When patients come in, we advise them to lose weight," said Dr. Richard E. Ostlund, Jr. "This paper suggests that more important than that is how the fat is distributed."

His study, conducted with healthy elderly people, found that body shape alone could account for a large portion of the differences in people's HDL cholesterol levels. Ostlund's study, conducted at Washington University School of Medicine, was published in the *New England Journal of Medicine*.

Women typically have higher HDL levels than men. As they grow older, women also tend to put on weight around the hips, while men are more prone to larger bellies.

Experts have long suspected that differences in sex hormones might explain the HDL disparity between men and women. However, the new study suggests that body shape, not sex, could be the key factor. It found that pear-shaped men tend to have high HDL, while apple-shaped women have lower HDL.

"It's not how fat you are; it's where the fat's located," said Ostlund. "The fat around your hips, the good fat that women have, is predominantly subcutaneous fat," or just underneath the skin. "But the fat you have in your belly is intra-abdominal fat. The difference is where the blood supply of those two areas drains."

Stomach fat surrounds the intestines, and its blood supply drains directly to the liver, he said. "The liver is sensitive to things that fat cells put out. The metabolism of the liver may be changed because of the intra-abdominal fat," including the liver's production of HDL. The blood from hip fat does not drain directly to the liver and so has less impact on the way it works, he said.

Ostlund's study was conducted on 77 men and 69 women, all in their 70s. To measure whether they were apples or pears, the researchers calculated the ratio of their waist-to-hip circumference. They found the ratio was the most powerful predictor of the HDL level, accounting for 32 percent of the variations.

Ostlund said dieting is a hard way to tackle the problem, since fat patterns may be established at birth. "It's very hard to change your waist-to-hip ratio," Ostlund said. "You can do it if you lose a massive amount of weight, but losing 10 to 20 pounds doesn't change it very much."

THE FAT DECADE

People are most likely to get fat between ages 25 and 34, and women face twice the risk, according to a decade-long study of nearly 10,000 adults.

The study, which monitored the weights of people ranging from age 24 to 74, said women ages 25 to 44 who began the study overweight gained the most weight of all subjects. Among 25- to 34-year-old women, blacks were 40 percent more likely than whites to gain a lot of weight. For women ages 35 to 44, blacks were 80 percent more likely to face a major weight gain, the researchers found.

As many as one-third of the 9,862 subjects were overweight when the study began. They were measured once between 1971 and 1975, and again between 1981 and 1984. Researchers led by epidemiologist David Williamson of the nutrition division at the U.S. Centers for Disease Control in Atlanta, defined a major weight gain as an increase of about 20 percent, or an estimated 30 pounds for a person of average height.

Among all women ages 25 to 44 who were overweight at the start, 14.2 percent experienced a major weight gain, compared with 5.6 percent among men of the same age. Among women of that age group who were of normal weight when the monitoring began, 6.2 percent gained a lot of weight, compared with 2.9 percent among men.

After age 55, weight levels in men and women studied began declining.

WOMEN, SMOKING, AND HEART ATTACKS

A woman who smokes is three times as likely as one who doesn't to have a heart attack, according to a Boston University study. Previous studies have found the same effect in men, but this was the first such study of women.

The study found that women who smoked more than 35 cigarettes a day had more than seven times the risk of a nonsmoker. But it also found that if a woman quits smoking, in three years her risk of a heart attack is no greater than that of someone who never smoked.

The Department of Health and Human Services (HHS) says heart disease is the leading cause of death in both sexes and the biggest cause in smoking-related deaths. In 1985, heart disease attributed to smoking killed 78,000 men and 37,000 women, according to HHS estimates.

Ronald M. Davis, director of the HHS Office on Smoking and Health, said, "We've known for many years that the benefits of quitting occur much more quickly for heart disease than for lung cancer and other cancers. If anything, this shows even more rapid benefits" for women who quit.

YOUNG MEN, SMOKING, AND CHOLESTEROL

Young men who smoke or have high cholesterol levels are more likely than others to show signs of heart disease before they reach age 35, according to a University of Chicago study.

Dr. Henry McGill said, "In this age group, smoking and cholesterol are about equally bad. What surprised me . . . was the effect of smoking."

The findings are based on autopsies of about 300 15- to 34-year-old white men who died violent deaths or in accidents. By age 34, one-fourth of the subjects already had what doctors called "raised lesions" in their arteries, representing the beginning of hardening of the arteries. Only one previous study had looked at hardening of the arteries in young people, McGill said.

McGill said a 25-year-old man who smoked and had high levels of good cholesterol would have twice the artery damage of a 25-year-old nonsmoker who had low levels of LDL.

CHOLESTEROL TEST ACCURACY

The accuracy of cholesterol screening tests varies widely, with portable testing machines used by poorly trained operators giving highly inaccurate results up to one-fourth of the time, according to researchers at the University of Minnesota School of Public Health.

They said poorly set instruments and inadequate training were mainly to blame for misleading readings, which can cause people to seek unneeded medical treatment or falsely reassure them they don't need it.

Michelle J. Naughton, a sociologist, said cholesterol screening results were within an acceptable range of accuracy in only one of four public screenings they analyzed. In the three other screenings, readings often strayed from true values by more than 14.2 percent, the largest range of error allowed under guidelines of the National Cholesterol Education Program, researchers said. True values were established on samples from the same subjects measured in a nationally standardized laboratory, they continued.

The highest rate of unacceptable results was 23.5 percent, among tests done by a cholesterol-screening company at an unidentified worksite, the researchers said. Other testing groups had rates of unacceptable error ranging from 6.9 percent, at a retail store; to 3.6 percent, at a grocery store; to zero percent, at the Minnesota State Fair, the researchers found.

Improve Your Health with These Important Books

Good Cholesterol, Bad Cholesterol by Eli Roth, M.D. and Sandra Streicher, R.N. .... paperback $8.95
Praised by experts as the finest book on cholesterol, this book covers every aspect of the cholesterol equation in a clearly understandable style. "A valuable guide into the benefits of a disease-preventive lifestyle." William C. DeVries, M.D.

Immune for Life by Arnold Fox, M.D. and Harry Fox, Ph.D. .... paperback $9.95
In the final analysis, most diseases are caused by a failure of the immune system to respond correctly. In *Immune for Life,* Dr. Fox shows the reader how to adopt a lifestyle that promotes a strong immune system, which he calls "our doctor within." Included is a program encompassing nutrition, mental attitude, and physical exercise.

Controlling High Blood Pressure edited by Franz H. H. Leenen, M.D. and R. Brian Haynes, M.D.
.... paperback $8.95
In this book, ten of North America's top hypertension specialists, each writing a chapter, cover every aspect of dealing with hypertension. Highly informative, comprehensive, and easy to understand.

Health-Related Cookbooks

Lean and Luscious, and *More Lean and Luscious* by Bobbie Hinman and Millie Snyder ...... each book $14.95
These two cookbooks each offer over 400 recipes. Each recipe is designed for today's low-fat, low cholesterol, high-fiber lifestyle. Each recipe comes with at-a-glance nutritional breakdown. Spiral comb-bound for easy reading.

Dairy Free Cookbook by Jane Zukin
.... hardcover $18.95
For people with little or no milk tolerance, this is a life saver. Included are recipes for both adults and children and guidelines for eating out. Recommended for gastro-enterologists, internists, and all who suffer from milk allergy or lactose deficiency.

FILL IN AND MAIL ... TODAY

PRIMA PUBLISHING
P.O. BOX 1260CAS
ROCKLIN, CA 95677

USE YOUR VISA/MC AND ORDER BY PHONE
(916) 624-5718 (M–F 9–4 PST)

Dear People at Prima,
I'd like to order the following titles:

Quantity	Title	Amount
_____	_____	_____
_____	_____	_____
_____	_____	_____
_____	_____	_____
_____	_____	_____

	Subtotal	$_____
	Postage & Handling	$ 3.00
	Sales Tax	$_____
	TOTAL (U.S. funds only)	$_____

☐ Check enclosed for $____ (payable to Prima Publishing)
Charge my ☐ MasterCard ☐ Visa

Account No. _____ Exp. Date _____

Signature _____

Your Name _____

Address _____

City/State/Zip _____

Daytime Telephone _____

YOU MUST BE SATISFIED, OR YOUR MONEY BACK!!!
Thank You for Your Order